I0122081

BEATING HISTAMINE INTOLERANCE NATURALLY

Dr. Scott A. Johnson

COPYRIGHT © 2024, by Scott A. Johnson

All Rights Reserved. No part of this publication may be reproduced or transmitted in any form or by any means, electronic or mechanical, including photocopying and recording, or introduced into any information storage and retrieval system without the written permission of the copyright owner. Brief quotations may be used in reviews prepared for magazines, blogs, newspapers, or broadcasts.

Beating histamine intolerance naturally / Scott A. Johnson

Cover design: Scott A. Johnson

Cover Copyright: © Scott A. Johnson 2024

ISBN-13: 979-8988720638

Published by Scott A. Johnson Professional Writing Services, LLC: Orem, UT

Discover more books by Scott A. Johnson at authorscott.com/shop

DISCLAIMERS OF WARRANTY AND LIMITATION OF LIABILITY

The author provides all information on an "as is" and "as available" basis and for informational purposes only. The author makes no representations or warranties of any kind, expressed or implied, as to the information, materials, or products mentioned. Every effort has been made to ensure accuracy and completeness of the information contained; however, it is not intended to replace any medical advice or to halt proper medical treatment, nor diagnose, treat, cure, or prevent any health condition or disease.

Always consult a qualified medical professional before using any dietary supplement or natural product, engaging in physical activity, or modifying your diet; and seek the advice of your physician with any questions you may have regarding any medical condition. Always consult your OB/GYN if you are pregnant or think you may become pregnant before using any dietary supplement or natural product, and to ensure you are healthy enough for exercise or any dietary modifications. The information contained in this book is for educational and informational purposes only, and it is not meant to replace medical advice, diagnosis, or treatment in any manner. Never delay or disregard professional medical advice. Use the information solely at your own risk; the author accepts no responsibility for the use thereof. This book is sold with the understanding that neither the author nor publisher shall be liable for any loss, injury, or harm allegedly arising from any information or suggestion in this book.

The Food and Drug Administration (FDA) has not evaluated the statements contained in this book. The information and materials are not meant to diagnose, prescribe, or treat any disease, condition, illness, or injury. You are encouraged to seek the most current information and medical care from your healthcare professional.

Contents

Histamine Intolerance Symptoms

Neurological (H2/H3)
Headache
Migraine
Brain fog
Sleep disorders
Dysregulated circadian rhythm
Anxiety
Dizziness
Vertigo
Tremors

Gastrointestinal(H1/H2/H3/H4)
Bloating
Fullness after eating
Diarrhea
Constipation
Flatulence
Stomach cramps
Acid reflux
Burning sensation
SIBO
SIFO
Leaky gut
Dysbiosis
Nausea
Vomiting

Musculoskeletal (H1/H2/H3/H4)
Muscle or joint pain
Fibromyalgia
Muscle twitches
Heavy legs

Systemic (H1/H2/H3/H4)
Chills
Flushes
Sweating
Difficulty regulating body temperature
Unexplained fatigue
Swelling
Listlessness

Ocular (H1/H2/H3/H4)
Eye swelling
Eye allergies
Glaucoma

Cardiovascular (H1/H2)
Low blood pressure
High blood pressure
Arrhythmia
Palpitations
Blood clots

Respiratory (H1/H2/H3)
Runny nose
Nasal congestion
Sneezing
Difficulty breathing
Asthma
Rhinitis
Constant throat clearing
Sore throat
Hoarseness
Postnasal drip

Skin (H1/H2/H4)
Itching
Rashes
Eczema
Hives
Acne

Urinary/Reproductive (H1/H2)
Urinary urgency
Frequent urination
Voiding difficulty
Incontinence
Menstrual cramps
Missed or irregular periods
Endometriosis
Estrogen dominance

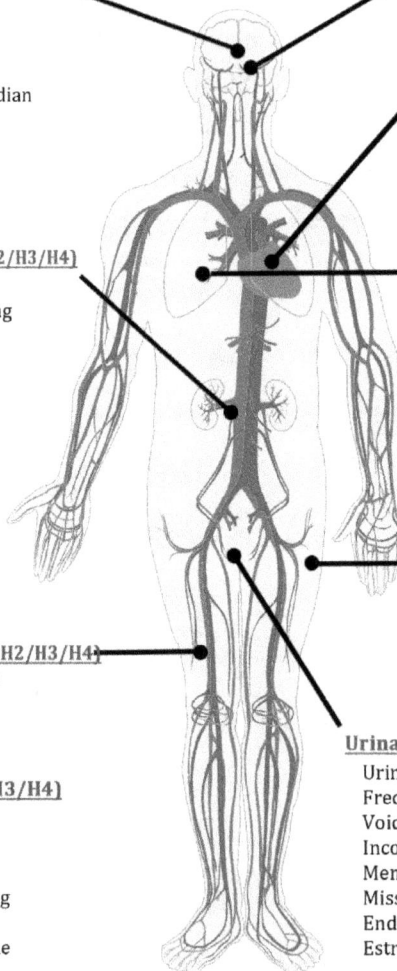

https://authorscott.com/shop/

1

WHAT IS HISTAMINE AND HISTAMINE INTOLERANCE?

Do you experience frequent headaches or migraines, persistent fatigue, unexplained muscle soreness, anxiety, attention deficit hyperactivity disorder (ADHD), recurrent gastrointestinal symptoms, or a constant need to clear your throat? What about an itchy tongue when you eat bananas, avocados, or sauerkraut? If you answered yes to one or more of these questions, then you may have histamine intolerance. What is histamine intolerance, and why could it be the origin of the above symptoms? To understand this, we first need to explore the basics of histamine and what it does.

The Diverse Role of Histamine in Human Health

Many people have heard of histamine and associate it with seasonal allergies. A plethora of antihistamine drugs are available over the counter for this exact purpose. But histamine is far more than a chemical that triggers allergies. It is a signaling chemical that your immune system releases to send messages between cells. It regulates the activity of other immune cells, such as T cells, B cells, monocytes, and dendritic cells. Histamine is a bioactive amine released in response to injury or infection, involved in the secretion of stomach acid, and acts as a neurotransmitter in the brain. So, it's clear that histamine is important for body functions when the appropriate amount is flowing through the body.

The Role of Mast Cells in Histamine Release and their Biological Function

Histamine is created inside immune cells called basophils, mast cells, and other cells (enterochromaffin cells, T cells, and keratinocytes). However, mast cells and basophils are the primary releasers of histamine because they store large quantities of histamine and quickly release them when stimulated. Found in connective tissue throughout our bodies, mast cells are frontline sentinels that defend against infections but have an opposing role in driving allergies. In response to a perceived threat—pathogens, allergens, injury, or other compounds—mast cells are activated, causing them to selectively or rapidly release mediating chemicals. Mast cells release a variety of immune system mediators, like histamine, heparin, and serotonin, and proteins and enzymes, such as cytokines and proteases, that trigger both rapid and long-term inflammation. This can lead to the classic allergy symptoms of nasal irritation, mucus production, watery eyes, and constricted airways. The reactions that follow mast cell responses are contingent on the tissue that is being affected by the threat.

Gastrointestinal response. When you eat something that is perceived as harmful, mast cells in the gut initiate a response that increases fluid secretion, promotes muscular contraction in the digestive system, and hastens peristalsis, which can trigger vomiting or diarrhea to quickly remove the threat from the body. What we see as symptoms of a condition are actually corrective actions being taken by the body to protect us against a threat—actual or perceived. Your body is attempting to remove the offending substance as quickly as possible to minimize harm and damage. Whether we experience allergies or healthy responses when faced with a perceived threat is determined by the balance of mast cells in the gastrointestinal tract and their activity. Mast cell overproduction or overactivation can cause a variety of gastrointestinal disorders—irritable bowel syndrome, upset stomach, cyclical or chronic nausea, and heartburn. Increased mast cell degranulation (the release of its granules and mediating chemicals) leads to excessive histamine in tissues, which can manifest as a wide variety of symptoms due to the actions of histamine on multiple cellular receptors and targets. Indeed, it can stimulate or hinder a variety of organs and systems, including the brain, skin, immune, reproductive, respiratory, and digestive systems.[1]

Mast cells also play an important role in maintaining a healthy gut microbiome. They are located throughout the lining of your gut, where they play an active role in destroying pathogenic bacteria. Fewer pathogenic bacteria means more space for healthy bacteria to thrive in the gut. Additionally, they serve to facilitate communication between the intestinal mucosa, gut microbiome, and the nervous system.[2] Indeed, the gut microbiome relies on a network of neurotransmitters (GABA, dopamine, serotonin) and neuromodulators (histamine) to facilitate communication between the enteric nervous system in the gut and the central nervous system. Signals created by these signaling molecules are transported to the central nervous system via the vagus nerve, and in response, the brain sends signals back via the vagus nerve that coordinates vital body functions. In this way, histamine acts as a communication hub to coordinate body systems' efforts to maintain health.

Respiratory response. In response to an inhaled threat, mast cells that line your respiratory tract constrict the airways and promote coughing, congestion, and increased mucus production. Smooth muscles in the airways relax or contract to control breathing. Histamine and other bronchoconstrictors exert their actions on the airways by increasing calcium ion concentrations in the smooth muscles of the airways, which stimulates a contractive response. Again, these are innate corrective responses your body takes to defend against and remove the offending substance. However, overactivation or overproduction of histamine can lead to respiratory conditions like asthma, chronic obstructive pulmonary disease, and even idiopathic pulmonary fibrosis. Mast cells must always be in balance to regulate their opposing roles of participating in the defense against respiratory infections without playing a pathogenic role in airway diseases.

Skin response. Mast cells are strategically located in the body at places where a high degree of contact with the host and the environment occurs, like the gastrointestinal tract, lungs, nasal passages, and the skin. They typically reside in the dermis, near blood vessels, nerves, and hair follicles.[3] Positioned in key locations, mast cells in the skin are well-equipped to defend against invading pathogens, respond to allergens, and interact with other immune cells that travel to locations of infection or injury. These interactions can be beneficial or harmful depending on whether the mast cells maintain balanced activity and histamine levels or overshoot. The characteristic actions of histamine in the skin include itching, swelling, redness, and inflammation.

Sometimes, threats that are ingested migrate from the digestive tract and into the bloodstream. As they circulate throughout the body, they are recognized by mast cells, including in the tissues of the skin. This leads to hives or a rash on the skin that may become chronic, like eczema.

The Role of Basophils in Immunity

Basophils are very similar to mast cells because they both are granulated cells—immune cells that contain specific granules in their cytoplasm that serve as immune regulators. Like mast cells, they create and release two chemicals (histamine and heparin) and lipid mediators (prostaglandins and leukotrienes) in response to immune threats. Histamine enlarges your blood vessels to improve blood flow, which allows more immune cells to quickly travel to, target, and respond to threats and heal affected tissues. Heparin prevents blood from clotting too quickly, thus thinning the blood and preventing blood clots from forming at the site of an injury or infection. Certain prostaglandins promote inflammation by widening blood vessels and increasing the permeability of capillaries. Doing so allows cells to migrate from the bloodstream to the site of injury or infection. Leukotrienes primarily function to recruit other immune cells (neutrophils) to areas of tissue damage and promote inflammation by producing cytokines. All these mediators are released to make necessary repairs to tissues and fight infections, but when they are released excessively in response to nonharmful substances, they can trigger allergic reactions.

Basophils can also indirectly attack threats by binding to B-cell white blood cells. By binding to these cells, the B cells release antibodies called immunoglobulin E (IgE), which has activity against pathogens and venoms.[4] Therefore, basophils are involved in immune defenses against pathogens, allergic responses, and blood clotting.

Histamine Metabolism

Histamine metabolism occurs by two primary pathways. Histamine N-methyltransferase (HNMT) is the first pathway by which histamine released by mast cells and basophils is metabolized and inactivated in the body. It is a protein found in the cytosol—the water-based fluid found within cells, as opposed to the cytoplasm that is present in the cell membrane—of cells in many tissues, such as the kidney, liver, spleen, ovaries, prostate, bronchi, trachea, and spinal cord.[5] HNMT involves methylation and produces *tele*-methylhistamine (t-MH). t-MH is further metabolized by monoamine oxidase B (MAO-B), producing tele-methylimidazole acetic acid (t-MIAA). The methylation of histamine is accelerated in the presence of methyl donors like S-adenosyl-L-methionine (SAMe).[6] A simple way to envision this process is to use the analogy of writing a report that you need to print. You initially type the report on your computer, producing an electronic document—the first phase, like when t-MH is produced. The next step is to send this electronic document to the printer (MAO-B) to be printed—producing a document on paper like when t-MIAA is produced from t-MH. Although a major histamine metabolism pathway, HNMT breaks down histamine to a lesser extent than the second pathway.

The second pathway involves oxidation via an enzymatic process. Enzymes are responsible for breaking down histamine so it doesn't build up in your body. Produced mainly in the kidneys, the thymus gland, and the intestinal lining of your digestive tract, diamine oxidase (DAO, also called histaminase) is an enzyme that serves the primary function of breaking down histamine in the body. It is found in high levels in the intestinal mucosa, strongly supporting the assertion that histamine intolerance originates in the gut. After oxidizing histamine, imidazole acetic acid is produced, which is further broken down by a group of enzymes known as aldehyde dehydrogenases. DAO takes the lead in histamine metabolism in the intestine and is continually secreted by the intestinal lumen.

Histamine intolerance is characterized by reduced DAO activity or the absence of the enzyme due to drug interactions, gene-related insufficiencies, or changes in the gut microbiome. Additionally, the consumption of certain histamine-rich foods can contribute to histamine intolerance by increasing the amount of histamine in the bloodstream.

Medications that May Trigger or Exacerbate Histamine Intolerance Symptoms

A variety of medications may trigger or exacerbate histamine intolerance symptoms due to their effects of increasing histamine or the inhibition of DAO activity.[7,8,9] Common medications that can do this include analgesics (NSAIDs, aspirin, morphine), antibiotics, high blood pressure drugs (verapamil, alprenolol, dihydralazine), muscle relaxants (pancuronium, alcuronium, D-tubocurarine), and motility agents (metoclopramide).[10] This is not a comprehensive list of all drugs capable of inhibiting DAO activity, but lists the most common drugs. Interestingly, vitamin C (ascorbic acid) and thiamine may also contribute to symptoms by reducing DAO activity, according to preclinical research.[11,12] Whether this translates to humans is debatable since vitamin C is frequently used to reduce histamine-related allergies and other research shows that it acts as an antihistamine.[13] If you are taking any of the aforementioned drugs, the offending drug, or drugs, need to be discontinued to reduce their interference with histamine metabolism.

Genetic Mutations Associated with Histamine Intolerance

Single nucleotide polymorphisms (SNPs) in any of the enzymes involved in histamine metabolism can interfere with the breakdown and elimination of histamine and the products of its catabolism. Methylenetetrahydrofolate reductase (MTHFR) is one of the most common mutations that people may experience, affecting about half of the human population. The MTHFR gene creates the MTHFR enzyme responsible for converting homocysteine into methionine and plays a vital role in methylation and detoxification as well. Methylation is important for optimizing DNA function, repairing damaged cells, processing hormones, balancing neurotransmitter levels, and metabolizing B vitamins. Undoubtedly, MTHFR and methylation are essential for all areas of health, and mutations in this critical gene can lead to allergies, hormonal dysregulation, mental health issues, sleep troubles, and histamine intolerance.

So, how are MTHFR mutations linked to histamine intolerance? Going back to earlier, HNMT is vital to metabolizing histamine and relies on the cofactor SAMe. MTHFR mutations cause lower MTHFR function, which disrupts HNMT's ability to process histamine. Eventually, this slower removal of histamine from the body triggers an array of symptoms associated with excess histamine levels. Furthermore, deficient methylation caused by MTHFR mutations hinders detoxification, leading to an inability to efficiently remove toxins and creating a buildup of histamine. Too much histamine means multiple symptoms of histamine intolerance occur, including headaches or migraines, fatigue, anxiety, skin problems, digestive disturbances, and abnormal menstrual cycles.

Mutations in DAO/AOC1 (amine oxidase copper-containing 1), MAO, and HNMT may also occur, which further interferes with histamine removal and exacerbates histamine intolerance and its many symptoms. The AOC1 gene creates DAO to speed the degradation of amines, including histamine and putrescine. DAO mutations obviously impair the metabolism of histamine in the body since the enzyme can't do its job well. Not surprisingly, DAO mutations are linked to sensitivity to NSAIDs since individuals with these mutations poorly metabolize histamine, and NSAIDs further limit histamine metabolism.[14] Fibromyalgia has even been associated with AOC1 mutations.[15] MAO-

B mutations interfere with the metabolism of intermediate metabolites produced during the metabolism of histamine. These mutations can also lead to cardiovascular and neurological conditions because of their involvement in mitochondrial and neurotransmitter regulation.[16] HNMT mutations also disrupt the metabolism and excretion of histamine, leading to a symptom-producing buildup. Of note, HNMT mutations frequently occur in Chinese and Japanese individuals.[17] Genetic testing can reveal whether any of these mutations exist and guide the management of histamine intolerance.

Health Begins and Ends in the Gut

Health, both physical and mental/emotional, begins and ends in the gut. And gut health is largely dependent on a healthy gut microbiome. When populations of microbes living in the gut become imbalanced—a condition called dysbiosis—the gut microbiome can further contribute to excess histamine production.[18] A greater abundance of histamine-producing bacteria creates a gut environment favoring the accumulation of high histamine levels in the gut and the subsequent absorption into the bloodstream, leading to the symptoms of histamine intolerance. Gut microbiota can produce histamine as a byproduct, such as *Helicobacter pylori, Klebsiella aerogenes, Cetobacterium somerae, Fusobacterium ulcerans, F. ulcerans* A, *F. varium, F. varium* A.[19,20,21] Surprisingly, *Lactobacillus saerimneri* creates almost one hundred times more histamine when compared to *L. rhamnosus*.[22] Other pathogenic bacteria, like *Pseudomonas aeruginosa*, have evolved to sense histamine and its metabolites, which allows them to attract more bacteria to the area and increase their virulence.[23] Dysbiosis is frequently observed in people diagnosed with histamine intolerance.[24,25] Lastly, excess histamine in the gut may reduce the production of short-chain fatty acids by healthy bacteria in the gut, which are vital byproducts that dramatically influence overall health.[26] Clearly, a healthy gut microbiome must be restored and maintained to address histamine intolerance. Indeed, gut health issues can increase food sensitivities because your gut releases more histamine as a defense against these food sensitivities and the symptoms they trigger.

When dysbiosis is present, leaky gut is nearly always present as well, and this too has been observed in people with histamine intolerance based on elevated stool zonulin levels.[27] Zonulin is a protein that controls the permeability of tight junctions between cells in the gastrointestinal tract. The more zonulin in the gut, the more open these tight junctions become. The opening of these tight junctions is a normal and necessary state that exists for nutrients and other vital molecules to get in and out of the intestines. But when these tight junctions open too much, they allow larger molecules to enter the bloodstream and initiate harmful immune reactions. Once this happens, your body remains in a primed state to react to those proteins each time they enter the bloodstream. Gut integrity must be maintained to reduce the effects of dietary histamine because leaky gut allows histamine to enter the bloodstream and cause these immune reactions. For a comprehensive approach to overcoming these two contributing factors to histamine intolerance, you are invited to read this author's book *Heal the Gut, Heal the Immune System*.

SIBO As a Potential Root Cause of Histamine Intolerance

Small intestinal bacterial overgrowth (SIBO), parasites, and candida overgrowth are all underlying causes of histamine intolerance via the gut. SIBO is a bacterial imbalance in the gut, specifically the small intestine. A healthy balance of good and bad bacteria and good and bad fungi/yeast in the gut normally keep each other in check. But sometimes the bad outcompete the good, overwhelming the beneficial bacteria and shifting gut balance to one where digestive disturbances and systemic symptoms occur.

Your small intestine plays a pivotal role in the digestion process because it is the location of nutrient absorption. Around ninety percent of nutrients from the foods and beverages you consume are absorbed in the small intestine.[28] The middle part of your small intestine, known as the jejunum, absorbs the most nutrients—carbs, fats, proteins, minerals, and vitamins. This is where those tight junctions mentioned earlier are vital. The walls of your small intestine contain densely packed folds—called tight junctions—to boost its surface area and maximize the absorption of nutrients from the small intestine into your bloodstream. Once in the bloodstream, nutrients can travel to key areas of your body to be used for vital functions.

After being metabolized and absorbed, nutrients continue their journey through the gastrointestinal tract via wavelike contractions known as peristalsis. This pushes food from the small intestine to the large intestine, which contains trillions of microorganisms that make up your gut microbiome. Microbes in the gut further break down remaining food, eventually forming stool to be passed out of the rectum. While the small intestine does not contain the immense collection of microbes that the large intestine does, it does contain a limited number of microbes. The small number of microbes in the small intestine can increase if gastrointestinal motility—the speed with which food travels through the gastrointestinal tract—is altered.

Three primary types of SIBO exist based on the gas that the overgrown microbes in the small intestine produce: (1) hydrogen, (2) methane, and (3) hydrogen sulfide. Most of the time, the type of SIBO you have is determined by a noninvasive breath test that measures the type and amount of gas present in your small intestine. Rarely, a duodenal aspirate procedure is performed, where some of the fluid from your small intestine is collected to measure the type and amount of gases present there.

Hydrogen-dominant SIBO is the most common type of SIBO. This type is associated with excess serotonin production in the gut, which affects mood when outside the gut but regulates peristalsis when in the gut. Too much serotonin in the gut leads to the rapid transit of food through the digestive tract, leading to poor nutrient absorption, diarrhea, cramping, and bloating. Western medicine typically attacks hydrogen-dominant SIBO with an antibiotic, frequently rifaximin, metronidazole, amoxicillin, ciprofloxacin, or neomycin.

Methane-dominant SIBO is the second-most-common type and is driven by single-celled organisms called methanogens, which produce methane gas by leveraging the hydrogen gas and carbon dioxide present in the small intestine. Since hydrogen gas is necessary to produce methane gas, hydrogen- and methane-dominant SIBO frequently occur at the same time. Contrarily to hydrogen-dominant SIBO, methanogens slow the speed that food travels through the digestive tract, which can cause constipation. Given its slower transit, food sits in the small intestine for longer and ferments, causing you to absorb more calories. Since methanogens are not bacteria, an antibiotic is not entirely effective except for killing the hydrogen-producing bacteria that contribute to methane-dominant SIBO. Instead, an antibiotic is usually paired with a prokinetic agent that increases gut motility. Fasting for at least four hours between meals may also be suggested to increase your migrating motor complex, which sweeps bacteria from your digestive tract.

The third and least common type of SIBO is the hydrogen sulfide-dominant type. This gas, which has a rotten egg smell, is naturally present in your digestive tract and actually acts as an anti-inflammatory agent and helps repair the mucosal ling of the gastrointestinal tract when present in healthy quantities.[29] However, if excess hydrogen sulfide-producing bacteria are present in the small intestine, damage to your gut can occur. Hydrogen sulfide-dominant SIBO can cause diarrhea, damage to gut cells, increase gut or systemic inflammation, destabilize the protective mucus layer of the digestive tract, and increase immune activity.[30] Left untreated, it increases the risk of colon cancer, inflammatory bowel disease, compromised immune function, and mitochondrial damage. Unfortunately, traditional breath tests are unable to detect hydrogen sulfide gas, so determining this type remains very challenging. Standard treatment is not available for hydrogen sulfide-dominant SIBO, so your health professional may simply ask you to restrict foods and supplements containing significant sulfur content.

Symptoms of SIBO include bloating, abdominal pain, flatulence, diarrhea, constipation, nausea, belching, loss of appetite, weight changes, and fatigue. Left untreated, SIBO can cause malabsorption, nutrient deficiencies, irritable bowel syndrome, thyroid dysfunction, osteoporosis, and skin disorders.

Nearly half of people treated for SIBO with antibiotic therapy relapse weeks to months after treatment.[31] For these individuals, the overgrown microbe may need to be identified, and a more targeted antimicrobial may be used—the right antimicrobial for the right bug. Remember: antibiotics indiscriminately kill both bad and good bacteria, which means you are likely contributing to imbalance while eliminating the offending microbe. Instead, dietary and lifestyle modifications should be employed along with natural, more selective antimicrobials, immune-balancing solutions, and natural remedies to reduce gas production (e.g., enteric-coated peppermint oil, fennel essential oil, and ginger herb or essential oil). For detailed information on targeted antimicrobials and immune-balancing solutions, refer to this author's book *Heal the Gut, Heal the Immune System*.

The Link Between Parasites and Histamine Intolerance

Parasites can also wreak havoc in your gut, and since your gut is connected to everything in your body, they can trigger histamine overload. Parasites are organisms that live in, on, or with a host organism and harm it. The three main types of parasites are ectoparasites, helminths, and protozoans. Ectoparasites (e.g., ticks, fleas, mites, and lice) live on the exterior of their hosts and usually transmit infections from the skin into the bloodstream. Helminths, including flukes, tapeworms, and roundworms, are parasitic worms that usually reside in the digestive tract, anywhere from the stomach to the large intestine. Found in your intestines or blood and tissues, protozoans enter the body through ingesting contaminated food or water, through person-to-person contact, or through the bite of a carrier (vector). They include amoebas, ciliates, flagellates, and sporozoans. Parasites are largely a foreign concept in developed populations, but they are far more common than most people think. Hundreds of millions of people are infected and don't even know it because they have few to no symptoms.

Symptoms of parasitic infections depend on the parasite you are infected with, but in general, include nausea, diarrhea, gas, constipation, appetite changes, rectal itching, bad breath, chronic allergies, fatigue, anxiety, depression, confusion, weight loss, anemia, circles under the eyes, and weight loss. While controversial, some researchers theorize that antigens produced in response to specific parasitic infections interact with IgE on the surface of mast cells, which initiates their degranulation and the release of histamine.[32] Mast cells and IgE are critical components of innate (mast cells) and adaptive (mast cells and IgE) responses, and they both participate in defense against certain parasites.[33,34] To defend against parasites, mast cells secrete their mediators, including histamine, to produce an inflammatory and adaptive immune response.[35] Clearly, parasites can trigger mast cell activation as an immune defense against these invaders. Once active, mast cells increase in number and the degree of their release of mediators. Release of histamine, proteases, cytokines, and more occurs to control the parasitic infection. Some health professionals point the finger at *Blastocystis hominis* and *Dientamoeba fragilis* as leading parasites linked to higher histamine levels and drivers of histamine intolerance and mast-cell-activation syndrome. Black walnut (*Juglans nigra*) herb is among the most commonly used antiparasitic herbs if you are diagnosed with or feel parasites are contributing to your histamine intolerance. Follow the directions on the product label or those of your health professional.

Candida, Mold, and Histamine Intolerance

Candida is a fungus or yeast that is commonly found in small amounts throughout the body that can cause infections in the mouth, vagina, intestines, and skin. When it grows, candida makes and releases a plethora of toxins, including histamine. Your body also produces histamine in response to candida overgrowth, leading to massive increases in histamine levels.[36] Like SIBO, fungi must maintain a delicate balance to avoid causing harm. When fungi become overgrown in the small intestines, it is called small intestinal fungal overgrowth (SIFO). Common symptoms of SIFO include digestive issues, nutritional deficiencies, and food cravings. In severe cases, candida can leave the digestive tract and enter the bloodstream, causing systemic symptoms such as confusion, fatigue, mood swings, anxiety, depression, skin problems, headaches or migraines, rapid breathing or heart rate, fever, chills, low blood pressure, and joint or organ pain. This yeast also eats at your intestinal lining, promoting leaky gut. When *candida* cells die, they release endotoxins—uric acid, acetaldehyde, and ethanol—that significantly tax the liver and kidneys and further exacerbate symptoms.

Mold is the growth that some fungi can form in places with a lot of moisture. These formations contain tiny reproductive cells called mold spores that can be released into the environment and inhaled by humans. Mold allergies occur when your body overreacts to mold spores you've breathed in and are characterized by sneezing, runny or stuffy nose, watery or itchy eyes, itchy nose and throat, cough, or dry, scaly skin. Specific molds, such as *Stachybotrys* or *Aspergillus*, produce mycotoxins. Chemical and inflammatory reactions to mold can also occur when exposed to mycotoxins, which initiate a strong inflammatory response in the body. These types of reactions lead to systemic symptoms like cognitive troubles, unexplained or widespread pain, significant fatigue, numbness or tingling in the extremities, unexplained weight gain or loss, tinnitus, digestive disturbances, mood disruptions, a metallic taste in the mouth, excessive thirst, hair loss, or rashes. When you're exposed to more mold than your body can handle, types of molds that you are sensitive to, mycotoxins, or molds known to trigger health issues, it can lead to mold toxicity. Of note, mycotoxins are systemically bioavailable, meaning that regardless of the route of exposure, they can travel to multiple organs and systems.[37,38,39,40] When inhaled, mycotoxins disrupt the respiratory barrier and increase their capacity to invade other tissues. In the gut, they disrupt the microbiome, which eventually leads to leaky gut. Mold allergies and mold mycotoxins (biotoxins) are a serious risk factor for histamine intolerance.

Many Western health-care practitioners dismiss or overlook mold toxicity because it can produce symptoms that overlap with a variety of other chronic conditions. The first step in diagnosing a mold allergy or mold toxicity is to have a certified mold inspector evaluate your home. If mold is found in your environment, a home urine test kit can be used to measure metabolites of mold and mycotoxins as well as glutathione levels—glutathione is often depleted during mold exposure. However, these test kits have drawbacks, including false negatives or positives, the fact that not all toxins are tested, that test levels don't always correlate to symptom severity, and that they are not covered by insurance. As a confirmatory step, a specific (s)IgE to mold mixture (Mx1) can be a useful diagnostic marker to verify mold-associated respiratory symptoms.[41] Combined, clinical criteria and symptoms, verification of mold in the environment, and test results can be used to confirm a mold condition.

So, what is the connection between mold exposure and histamine intolerance? When mold spores are inhaled, they navigate your airways, where they are recognized by immune cells, including mast cells. Your immune system recognizes them as invaders and, in response, activates mast cells, which release histamine and other defensive mediators.[42] Mast cells also provoke increases in prostaglandin 2 levels, leading to hypersensitivity in multiple body systems. A cascade of inflammation keeps your immune system on high alert and sparks a constant influx of histamine that can lead to histamine intolerance. Mold toxicity is more likely to occur in individuals who already have a dysregulated immune system (autoimmune, autoinflammatory, immunodeficiency, allergies, etc.) because of the exacerbation of the preexisting immune dysfunction.[43] Addressing mold issues may be an important part of managing histamine intolerance on your path to better health.

Mitochondrial Function and Histamine Intolerance

Cellular metabolism is a complex process involving thousands of pathways. While we usually think of metabolism as simply digesting food, metabolism technically involves chemical reactions that take place inside cells. Thousands of chemical reactions are constantly carried out in cells to keep the cell healthy. Healthy cells lead to healthy tissues and organs and, ultimately, a healthy body. These chemical reactions are intrinsically linked to metabolic pathways. Cells rely on a continual flow of energy to fuel the energy-requiring chemical reactions that they perform.

Most people know that the mitochondria inside cells act as the powerhouse of the cell (bioenergetics). However, their function goes far beyond the conversion of nutrients to energy as they make multifaceted contributions to cellular metabolism. Mitochondria coordinate cellular adaptation to stressors, such as DNA damage, oxidative stress, and nutrient scarcity.[44] They also produce the raw materials for the production of functional products (DNA, RNA) and macromolecules (lipids, proteins). Indispensable in the management of cellular waste, mitochondria repurpose cellular waste—hydrogen sulfide, ammonia, lactate, reactive oxygen species—that researchers now recognize play functional roles in human health.[45] Thinking back to our SIBO discussion, their role in lowering hydrogen sulfide levels by oxidizing it to ultimately create sulfate, mitochondrial support may be important for hydrogen sulfide-dominant SIBO. In addition, they store calcium for cell signaling, create heat, and help regulate cellular growth and death. Obviously, maintaining healthy mitochondrial function is crucial for overall cellular health and total health.

Mitochondrial function is central to cellular metabolism and cellular resilience. Without healthy cellular metabolism and resilience, your cells stay in defense mode and are unable to restore and maintain healthy function. Think of it this way. If you're in a dodgeball game and you are the only person left on your team facing ten members of the other team, and they have all of the balls, you would be completely in defense mode. You could be targeted and hit by a ball from a variety of sources that keep your focus on defense. However, if you were in a situation where there were ten individuals left in the game, five on each team, some of you could focus on defense while others could go on the offensive. Your cells require similar support and numbers to participate in the essential restoration and maintenance of cellular processes.

Another important factor in mitochondrial function is a process called mitophagy. Mitophagy is a cellular process that removes or recycles dysfunctional, damaged, or unnecessary mitochondria to fine-tune mitochondrial numbers and preserve energy metabolism. It also regulates the mitochondrial biogenesis of new, fully functional mitochondria. Fundamentally, mitophagy is a quality control mechanism that serves to maintain cellular homeostasis. Impaired mitophagy negatively affects cellular health and contributes to age-related chronic conditions—neurodegenerative conditions, cardiovascular disease, and cancer—making maintaining healthy mitophagy vital for cellular and human health.[46] Therapeutic interventions that stimulate mitophagy may mitigate these age-related chronic conditions.

More recently, evidence indicates that mitochondria are actively involved in mast cell activation.[47] When an antigen enters the body and stimulates a mast cell response, it is accompanied by mitochondrial fragmentation—mitochondrial fission, the process where mitochondria divide into two separate mitochondrial organelles—and then secreted as an important first step in the release of mast cell mediators, including histamine.[48] Mitochondria play an important role in regulating cell signaling within the immune system, and defects in mitochondrial function play an important role in pathways that lead to allergic responses.[49] Without healthy mitochondrial function, histamine is likely to build up in the body to levels sufficient to initiate histamine-related symptoms. This emerging evidence demonstrates the mitochondria are actively involved in many stages of mast cell activation and may play a role in histamine intolerance.

The Importance of Nutrition in Relation to Histamine Intolerance

Food quality matters, and most whole foods are lower in histamine. Whenever possible, eat local, fresh, and in-season foods. Histamine from foods is absorbed through the gut lining. The shield against excess absorption of dietary histamine in the bloodstream is maintaining optimal DAO levels and activity. In addition, certain foods are known to contain higher histamine levels or trigger the release of histamine and should be strictly limited or avoided.

- Tomatoes
- Tomatillo
- Chlorella
- Spirulina
- Kelp
- Seaweed
- Potatoes
- Aged cheeses
- Beans
- Peanuts
- Walnuts
- Cured deli meats
- Dry-fermented sausages
- Chocolate and cacao
- Citrus fruits
- Pineapple
- Strawberries
- Bananas
- Dried fruit
- Papaya
- Avocados
- Peppers
- Spinach
- Kale
- Arugula
- Cauliflower
- Broccoli
- Butternut squash
- Spaghetti squash
- Eggplant
- Fermented foods
- Pickled and canned foods (particularly canned fish)
- Vinegar-containing foods
- Smoked fish
- Shellfish
- Cow's milk
- Beer
- Red wine
- Rice vinegar
- Wheat germ
- Artificial dyes and preservatives
- Processed foods

In addition to the above, some foods or beverages may block DAO activity.

- Alcohol
- Energy drinks
- Tea (green, black, mate)

Beyond the list of "don'ts," there are many foods that are beneficial and you should enjoy on a regular basis if you have histamine intolerance.

- Grass-fed-and-finished beef
- Free-range organic poultry
- Wild-caught fish
- Cooked eggs
- White rice
- Quinoa
- Millet
- Amaranth
- Almond milk
- Rice milk
- Coconut milk
- Olive oil
- Coconut oil
- Natural peanut butter
- Apple
- Apricot
- Pear
- Grapes
- Blueberries
- Blackberries
- Cherries
- Mango
- Kiwi
- Watermelon
- Fresh vegetables (except spinach and eggplant)
- Leafy herbs

Remember, though, that each person is unique, and this biological uniqueness means that each person also has an individual threshold of tolerance. Many people with histamine intolerance can eat most low-histamine foods, a serving of moderate-histamine foods, and only very small amounts of high-histamine foods daily. Foods very high in histamine are rarely tolerated. Start by eliminating one food for about two weeks. Blood tests and/or food challenges are also an option. As you improve your health, your histamine tolerance level will also increase, and symptoms diminish.

Signs and Symptoms of Histamine Intolerance

The clinical manifestations, or symptoms, of histamine intolerance consist of a wide range of gastrointestinal and systemic symptoms. These diverse symptoms occur due to interaction with four histamine receptors (H1, H2, H3, H4) distributed in different organs and tissues of the body that activate signaling pathways when histamine attaches to them. H1 receptors are located throughout the body, including neurons, smooth muscle airway cells, and blood vessels, and are associated with allergic responses. Activation of these receptors by histamine binding causes the stereotypical allergic or anaphylactic reactions: itching, pain, vasodilation, low blood pressure, irregular heartbeat, flushing, and airway constriction. H1 receptors are also involved in regulating the sleep-wake cycle, body temperature control, food intake, emotional responses, aggressive behavior, memory, and learning.[50] The H1 receptor is a major target for allergic reactions.

Found mostly in the gastric mucosa, smooth muscle cells, and heart, activation of H2 receptors primarily regulates gastric acid secretion. They are also involved in vascular permeability, decrease blood pressure, cause flushing, promote headaches, elevate heart rate, and induce airway constriction. H2 receptors are a target in the treatment of duodenal ulcers.

H3 receptors are primarily found in neurons involved in the histamine system (histaminergic—mostly the central nervous system and, to a lesser extent, the peripheral nervous system) and involved in neurotransmitter release and balance. Specifically, they moderate the release and levels of histamine, dopamine, serotonin, noradrenaline, and acetylcholine in the central nervous system. Activation of H3 receptors can also interfere with neurological control of blood vessel constriction in the nasal mucosa, which would normally narrow the nasal passages in response to an inhaled threat. They are attractive targets for the treatment of cognitive disorders because of their involvement in neurotransmitter equilibrium.

Present in bone marrow cells and stem cells (peripheral hematopoietic cells), H4 receptors play important roles in immune function. They regulate eosinophil migration and the recruitment of mast cells, leading to the amplification of immune responses controlled by histamine and, eventually, to chronic inflammation.[51] They are also involved in T cell differentiation. H4 receptors are considered promising targets for autoimmune and inflammatory disorders because of their roles in immune responses and chronic inflammation.

Adverse reactions associated with histamine intolerance are complex and often affect multiple different organ systems. Research suggests that the most common symptoms of histamine intolerance are gastrointestinal bloating (92%), fullness after a meal (73%), diarrhea (71%), abdominal pain (68%), and constipation (55%).[52] Other symptoms reported by people with histamine intolerance included a burning sensation in the mouth, tongue, or anus; migraine; shaking or heavy legs; weakness; leg swelling; listlessness; fatigue; insomnia; poor concentration; heartburn; dry skin; eye inflammation; anxiety; difficulty breathing; sore throat; hoarseness; abnormal heartbeat; and high blood pressure. Complicating the picture, almost all people (97%) with histamine intolerance reported three or more symptoms involving different organs, with an average of eleven symptoms per person. Because symptoms are nonspecific and manifest in varied ways, there is a lack of consensus on what should define clinical histamine intolerance.

Although gastrointestinal symptoms appear to be the most common signs of histamine intolerance, other body systems can also be affected due to the ubiquitous presence of histamine receptors throughout the human body. Respiratory symptoms may include nasal congestion and discharge, sneezing, coughing, asthma, sore throat, and labored breathing. Skin symptoms comprise itching, swelling, flushing, hives, and eczema. Manifestations in the cardiovascular system, such as low or high blood pressure and rapid heart rate, are less frequent. Anxiety, headache or migraine, vertigo, dizziness, insomnia, fatigue, and poor concentration occur when the nervous system is affected. Musculoskeletal system manifestations include muscle twitches, muscle pain, fibromyalgia, and joint pain. Menstrual cramps, irregular periods, endometriosis, and estrogen dominance are potential reproductive signs of histamine intolerance. More recently, lower urinary tract symptoms, such as urgency, frequency, voiding difficulty, and incontinence, have been associated with histamine intolerance, with 88 percent of those manifesting with urinary tract symptoms having at least one SNP—AOC1 SNPs being linked to the most severe symptoms.[53] As mentioned above, whole-body symptoms like fatigue and listlessness may also occur. Symptoms vary widely and can be incredibly vague because histamine can initiate an inflammatory response in so many parts of the body.

Hope to Beat Histamine Intolerance Naturally

With a better understanding of the role of histamine in health and the symptoms of histamine intolerance, you're ready to move on to the next chapter, which is diagnosing it. It will help your health-care professional if you have a detailed list of your symptoms, things that improve or exacerbate these symptoms, any medications or supplements you are using currently, and a health history. One of the most important things is to maintain hope. There is power in hope; and histamine intolerance can be addressed when the appropriate strategies are employed.

2

DIAGNOSING HISTAMINE INTOLERANCE

Despite significant advances in the understanding of histamine intolerance, the clinical diagnosis of histamine intolerance remains challenging. A lack of validated and reliable diagnostics tests combined with widely varying symptoms that overlap with other conditions often means that histamine intolerance is diagnosed by a process of elimination. This is especially true since DAO levels in the bloodstream don't necessarily correlate with DAO activity in the gut.[54] However, DAO deficiency is commonly observed in people presenting with various symptoms of histamine intolerance—up to 88 percent of people.[55,56,57,58,59] Further obscuring diagnosis is the observation that many individuals without histamine intolerance randomly react in the histamine provocation test and no relationship between the ingestion of histamine-containing foods and individual symptoms can be consistently established.[60,61] The combination of diagnostic criteria currently used involves the appearance of typical symptoms, the exclusion of other related disorders, trial dietary modifications, and the performance of complementary tests.

Medical History, Symptoms Assessment, and Skin-prick Tests

A medical history involving the assessment of symptoms is the first step. If two or more symptoms of histamine intolerance are present, ruling out related disorders and potential causes of increased plasma histamine is required. Food allergies should be considered via a skin-prick test and systemic mastocytosis (abnormal levels or activity of mast cells in the body) with a tryptase test. Skin-prick tests involve pricking your skin and inserting a small amount of a potential allergen while monitoring your body's response. If you're potentially allergic to the substance, a reddish, elevated bump with a red ring will appear. The fifty-skin-prick test has emerged as a possible tool to diagnose histamine intolerance since 79 percent of people with histamine intolerance present with a histamine wheal greater than or equal to three millimeters after fifty minutes, as opposed to only 18.7 percent of people without histamine intolerance.[62] However, a response to a substance topically on the skin does not necessarily correlate to an allergic response when ingested. Moreover, a skin-prick test may show negative results for all substances except for a strong reaction to the positive control. On the opposite side of this, skin-prick tests are significantly susceptible to false positives as well. Further assessment through an IgE immunoassay should occur due to skin-prick test limitations. IgE immunoassays measure levels of food-specific IgE (sIgE) in the blood. Values have been established for many common food allergies that correspond to a ninety-five percent accuracy. Supervised food challenges may also be required. However, people presenting with food intolerance are typically negative in both the skin-prick testing and food-specific IgE immunoassays.[63] As you can tell, diagnosing histamine intolerance requires great patience and perseverance.

Differential Diagnosis: Exclusion of Food Allergies, Cross-reactions, and Nonallergic Reactions

The exclusion of other possible causes, such as genuine food allergy, cross-reactions, and nonallergic reactions (fructose malabsorption, lactose intolerance, sorbitol malabsorption), called a differential diagnosis, is of utmost importance. Gastrointestinal disorders that can trigger DAO deficiency should also be ruled out. These conditions include colorectal cancer, celiac disease, and carbohydrate malabsorption. Moreover, certain chronic infections, such as *Pseudomonas aeruginosa* or *Mycoplasma pulmonis* airway infections, may increase histamine levels in the body. Histamine intolerance may coexist with, or be a result of, these conditions.

Ruling Out DAO-Inhibiting Medications

Another factor is to determine if any drugs you are taking may be DAO inhibitors. Review the previous list of common drugs that decrease DAO activity and talk to your health-care professional about other drugs that could potentially be contributing to or the cause of your histamine intolerance symptoms. If any offending drugs are identified, alternatives should be explored.

A Low-histamine Diet

Limitation of histamine in the diet is the next exclusionary step in diagnosis. Ideally, a low-histamine diet should be followed for four to eight weeks. However, implementing a low-histamine diet for just two weeks combined with the support of a DAO supplement with meals is also effective. If histamine is a challenge, symptomatic relief should occur during this two-week trial. Journaling of all food and beverage consumption and documentation of any symptoms felt during the day, including the time they occurred, is also necessary. The following foods are usually avoided while on this diet: fermented dairy products, cheese, fermented vegetables, pickles or pickled vegetables, kombucha, cured or fermented meats, wine, beer, alcohol, champagne, fermented soy products, tomatoes, ketchup, eggplant, spinach, frozen, salted, or canned fish, and vinegar. Additionally, highly processed junk foods should be avoided, and fresh, local foods should be emphasized. Typically, symptoms of histamine intolerance begin between thirty minutes and a few hours after eating a symptom-provoking food. If remission or improvement of symptoms is noticed while on this diet, further complementary tests are warranted.

Measuring DAO Enzyme Activity

The determination of DAO enzyme activity can be accomplished through a blood (serum) test or intestinal biopsy. A serum test is far less invasive and can be a useful diagnostics tool, together with a detailed medical history, to differentiate histamine intolerance and food allergy.[64] Intestinal biopsy through gastroscopy can be a highly sensitive diagnostics tool to evaluate DAO activity in the intestines if warranted.

Laboratory	Plasma Histamine	Total IgE	Diamine Oxidase	Histamine Urinary Excretion – 24h
LabCorp	0.3-1.0 ng/mL	6-495 IU/mL		
Quest Diagnostics	<1.8 ng/mL	<114 kU/L		
Precision Point Diagnostics	<1.2 ng/mL		>42 ng/mL	
ARUP Laboratories	0-8 nmol/L	<215 kU/L		0-60 mcg/L/day
Sciotec			>80 HDU/mL	
NIH			>10 ng/mL	

Measuring Lipopolysaccharide Production

Another confirmatory test for histamine intolerance is to measure lipopolysaccharide (LPS) production. Histamine triggers the production of prostaglandins and interleukins by LPS via activating H1 receptors, which further upregulates the expression and function of H1 receptors and intensifies histamine-provoked inflammatory responses.[65] This links LPS production to histamine receptor activity and suggests they play a role in regulating histamine signaling.

Distinguishing Mast Cell Activation Syndrome and Histamine Intolerance

Histamine intolerance is often confused with mast-cell-activation syndrome (MCAS) because they both involve mast cells and present with similar symptoms. However, the difference is that with MCAS, mast cells release multiple chemical mediators, not just histamine, whereas mast cells release only histamine in true histamine intolerance. MCAS involves inflammation in multiple systems triggered by a variety of stimuli, like foods, hormones, stress, chemicals, pathogens, and electromagnetic frequencies. To make it more complicated, histamine intolerance can be an indicator of MCAS, actually a subset of MCAS, but it is not the only factor that would lead to an MCAS diagnosis. People with mild-moderate MCAS frequently have similar symptoms to people with histamine intolerance, whereas those with severe MCAS have a more definitive subset of symptoms.[66] The correlation between dietary factors and the onset of symptoms may be relevant in both histamine intolerance and MCAS. A comprehensive health history and labs are necessary to distinguish the two conditions.

Genetic Testing and Biomarkers of Histamine Metabolism

Two additional diagnostics tools that may be utilized are genetic testing for SNPs and the determination of biomarkers of histamine metabolism in urine and stool samples. SNPs can be evaluated from blood or oral mucosa samples and read in days to receive results. Currently, there are four different SNPs of the AOC1 gene linked to a higher risk of histamine intolerance.[67] Genetic testing of AOC1 genes is the most relevant to histamine intolerance diagnosis and can support the results of other diagnostics criteria. Other gene mutations that affect histamine intolerance include MTHFR, MAO, HNMT, histamine decarboxylase (HDC), and histamine receptor H1 (HRH1). As explained earlier, MTHFR mutations can disrupt HNMT's ability to process histamine and lead to a buildup of histamine in the body. Insufficient MAO or changes in the gene responsible for its production can reduce histamine metabolism and increase histamine concentrations in the body. Variations in the HNMT gene interfere with a histamine metabolism pathway and increase histamine levels. The HDC gene provides instructions for creating the histidine decarboxylase enzyme, which converts dietary histidine into histamine. Mutations in this gene can either decrease or increase histamine production depending on the variation. Lastly, HRH1 is a gene involved in the regulation of how sensitive your H1 receptors are to histamine. Mutations in this gene can increase H1 receptor responses to histamine-exacerbating symptoms by heightening sensitivity or reducing sensitivity and impairing H1 receptor function and responses. While genetics can play a role in histamine intolerance, simply having a mutation in one of these genes doesn't mean you are doomed to have histamine intolerance. Genes require triggers to set them off, such as dietary, environmental, and lifestyle factors. A comprehensive approach that considers all the factors involved in histamine intolerance symptoms is imperative to managing it.

People with histamine intolerance have a distinct urinary profile with lower levels of 1-methylhistamine (MHA; also n-methylhistamine).[68,69] The reference range for urinary 1-methylhistamine varies according to age, as follows: age 0–5 years—120–510 mcg/g creatinine, age 6–16 years—70–330 mcg/g creatinine, and age 17+ years—30–200 mcg/g creatinine. Given it is less invasive than blood draws and intestinal biopsies, urinalysis may be a preferred method to diagnose histamine intolerance, especially in children. Basic stool tests analyze histamine levels in your poop. Even more important would be a GI-Map Stool Test to analyze your gut microbiome. This test can determine the presence and levels of histamine producers in your gut, such as *Morganella, Klebsiella, Pseudomonas, Proteus,* and *Citrobacter freundii*. High levels of these bacteria suggest that histamine intolerance is rooted in the gut, and gut support is vital to healing. Another stool test is the advanced intestinal barrier assessment, which directly measures DAO and histamine levels as well as gut integrity. It provides a histamine-to-DAO ratio to reveal whether you have the proper balance between histamine and DAO to metabolize it. One last stool test is the GI Effects Comprehensive Profile. This one- or three-day collection test evaluates intestinal inflammation, digestive function, and the gut microbiome. It provides insights into the bacteria present in the gut and is helpful for diagnosing irritable bowel syndrome and inflammatory bowel disease.

Trial and Error and Lots of Patience

Trial and error are inherently involved in diagnosing histamine intolerance. Be patient with your health-care professional and yourself as you perform the right tests and try the necessary solutions to correctly diagnose histamine intolerance. For many health-care practitioners, they are learning what works best alongside you.

3

THE THREEFOLD APPROACH TO EFFECTIVELY MANAGING HISTAMINE INTOLERANCE: DECREASE HISTAMINE INPUT

To effectively manage histamine intolerance, the focus must be threefold: (1) decrease dietary histamine; (2) improve histamine metabolism, particularly DAO activity; and (3) promote cellular health and metabolism to reduce cellular histamine release. Addressing gut health and genetic polymorphisms are factors tackled as part of poor histamine metabolism.[70,71] It is important that you understand that no amount of supplementation is going to overcome a high-histamine diet. So, dietary modifications are essential to defeat histamine intolerance.

Reduce Histamine Input and Production

To reduce dietary histamine, refer to the lists of foods that are high in histamine. These foods should be limited or removed from your diet completely. Shift foods to those lower in histamine, such as fresh beef, fresh fish (hake, trout, plaice), fresh chicken, eggs, fresh fruit (with the exception of tomatoes, tomatillos, avocados, citrus fruits, pineapple, strawberries, bananas, peppers, and dried fruit), fresh vegetables (except eggplant, spinach, kale, arugula, broccoli, cauliflower, certain squash, and potatoes), milk substitutes (preferably homemade), and herbal teas. Based on surveys that ask people with histamine intolerance which foods trigger symptoms, there is a list of so-called histamine liberators, or foods that are low in histamine but which may trigger the release of histamine from mast cells and basophils. These include instant foods, grapes, bananas, citrus fruits, strawberries, seafood, papaya, spinach, pineapples, chocolate, nuts, wine, and green tea.[72] One answer as to why these foods may spark symptoms of histamine intolerance despite being low in or devoid of histamine is the interference of histamine metabolism by other competing amines. One study found exactly this: that the amines putrescine and cadaverine significantly delayed histamine degradation even at low concentrations.[73] Like histamine, these dietary amines are found in many foods, such as fish, fish products, fermented foods, and cheese.[74] Other amines—tyramine, spermidine, and spermine—only inhibited histamine degradation at the highest concentrations tested, meaning that you would likely need to eat a lot of them to experience symptoms. Tyramine is found in alcohol, cured and processed meat, aspartame, monosodium glutamate (MSG), coffee, chocolate, soy sauce, pickled fish, aged cheeses, bananas, grapes, citrus fruits, and avocados. Foods highest in spermidine include wheatgerm, soybeans, mature cheeses, mushrooms, peas, chicken liver, beef, mangos, broccoli, cauliflower, and hazelnuts. Vegetables and meat products are high in spermine, as are aged cheeses. Some health professionals and researchers consider the concept of histamine liberators as an unproven theory with little merit despite this research suggesting a possible mechanism of action. Despite this, these reactions to foods are based on the actual experience of individuals who have histamine intolerance, so this concept cannot be discounted entirely.

Get Seven to Nine Hours of Restful Sleep Per Night

In addition to dietary adjustments, focusing on other lifestyle factors can also improve histamine intolerance symptoms. Inadequate or nonrestful sleep can be signs of histamine intolerance. At the same time, getting seven to nine hours of restful sleep per night is vital for managing histamine intolerance and overall health. Histamine plays a major role in regulating our internal clock, or circadian rhythm. Histamine receptors are found throughout your body, and this includes the hypothalamus, which exerts its effects on all major regions of the central nervous system. Inhibiting H1 receptors promotes sleep while activating H1 receptors keeps you awake. H3 receptors are similarly involved in sleep and wakefulness. Histamine neurons are generally more active during periods of wakefulness, while they are inactive during sleep. Animal models have even found that histamine stabilizes sleep-wake states, providing a rigid structure to the various stages of sleep. The researchers found that mice lacking histamine experienced more REM sleep and jumped more frequently between sleep and wake states.[75] Histamine worked together with orexin to regulate wakefulness and was more involved in activating cortical regions of the brain. Knowing this, histamine can be considered a wakefulness-promoting substance and sleep-wake stabilizer, especially when you consider it in the context of the drowsiness caused by antihistamines.

Your body naturally releases the most histamine at around 3:00 a.m., so your body histamine is at its highest between the hours of 3:00 a.m. and 5:30 a.m.[76] To understand how this affects sleep, we need to use the analogy of a bathtub. We'll call it your "histamine bathtub." Imagine you want to take a warm bath. You fill the tub with warm water to your desired level. Under normal circumstances, you would now shut off the faucet to prevent overflowing the tub. However, in the case of histamine intolerance, your faucet malfunctions, and you are not able to shut off the faucet, thus overfilling your histamine bathtub. Eventually, this causes the water to flow out of the tub, and damage to the home can occur. The warm water represents your body's release of histamine, and the bathtub represents your body's capacity to manage histamine. Your bathtub drain is like your DAO enzyme. As long as it is not clogged (suppressed DAO activity), your body can let out water to avoid an overflow condition. But if you have histamine intolerance, your drain is clogged, and the faucet is stuck open, creating histamine overflow. So, when your body releases histamine at 3:00 a.m. into an already full bathtub, because you have histamine intolerance and an already full histamine bathtub, it excites your brain and can cause you to wake up.

While you work to decrease the histamine in your bucket, practice good sleep hygiene. Consider taking 0.5 to 1 mg of melatonin or tart cherry extract that naturally contains small amounts of melatonin. And don't forget to diffuse sleep-supporting essential oils like lavender, vetiver, cedarwood, and sweet orange.

TART CHERRY EXTRACT (Montmorency; contains about 13 ng melatonin/g of extract)	
Typical dose	30–60 mL of juice, half hour before bed; Capsules/softgels as instructed on the product label
Cautions and contraindications	Pregnancy, lactation
Interactions	None currently known
Potential adverse effects	Well tolerated, upset stomach, loose stools

Reduce Toxic Load

Reduce your toxic load and support your body's natural detoxification and elimination channels. Drink purified water. Choose natural personal care, household, and beauty products that limit your exposure to toxins. Avoid BPA plastics and substitute bamboo, wood, organic cotton, and other natural alternatives instead. Eat organic foods whenever possible. Move often in an enjoyable type of physical activity. Consider using an infrared sauna on a regular basis. Lastly, aid detoxification through the use of fulvic acid and humic acid.

A product of decomposition and formed through geochemical and biological reactions, fulvic acid acts as a voracious binder of toxins and heavy metals to neutralize them and safely escort them from the body without also escorting important vitamins, minerals, and nutrients from the body. Its unique chemical structure allows it to bind to heavy metals, forming stable, soluble complexes that can be easily excreted in the urine. Think of fulvic acid as your personal bodyguard. When he notices a potential threat in your home (body), he puts the threat in handcuffs attached to his own wrist and forcefully directs the threat to the nearest exit without escorting family members (beneficial nutrients) from the house. Even though fulvic acid has a small molecular size, it can bind many times its weight, which makes it an excellent carrier of both nutrients (to deliver to cells) and toxins (to escort out of the body).

In addition, fulvic acid improves the permeability of cell membranes to support the efficient exchange of nutrients and waste products at the cellular level. In other words, it acts as a gatekeeper to eliminate toxins from inside the cell and allow the passage of vital nutrients into the cell. Because it is alkalizing in nature, it helps maintain balanced body pH levels. It also has nutritional value, providing magnesium, zinc, calcium, and dozens of trace minerals in readily absorbable forms. Fulvic acid is a natural electrolyte because it contains essential ions like sodium, chloride, and potassium.

Like fulvic acid, humic acid is a decomposition product. Fulvic acid is actually a component of humic acid. Humic acid differs in its color, molecular weight, acidity, polymerization capacity, and carbon and oxygen content. Specifically, it is formed from the decay of prehistoric life through a process called humification. It, too, acts as a binder for toxins and heavy metals but tends to stay in the gastrointestinal tract, whereas fulvic acid is capable of cellular detoxification due to its smaller size. In addition, humic acid has significant positive effects on the gut microbiome.[77] Lastly, both fulvic acid and humic acid have shown the ability to bind to glyphosate in water, suggesting that they may also help the body eliminate this highly toxic pesticide from the body.[78] Detoxifying the body of glyphosate is critical to overall health because it is found nearly ubiquitously in humans due to its extensive use in agriculture globally.[79] Glyphosate compromises the tight junctions in your gut, allowing it and other larger molecules to leave the gut and trigger immune reactions in the body.[80] Specifically, glyphosate increases the expression of interleukin 33 (IL-33), which is involved in T helper type 2 (Th2)- and IgE-mediated histamine release from mast cells.[81] This suggests that glyphosate may ignite an immune cascade that amplifies mast cell activity and contributes to histamine overload. It also disrupts gut microbiome balance, shifting microflora to favor an overgrowth of pathogens.[82] Anything that can help eliminate glyphosate from the body and therefore reduce its harmful effects is positive for human health.

Before supplementing with fulvic or humic acid, you should choose a high-quality supplement that contains both fulvic acid and humic acid. These two organic acids are naturally found together, and taking them together provides some unique benefits.

FULVIC ACID with HUMIC ACID (Or Fulvic Acid 400X)	
Typical dose	As instructed on the product label
Cautions and contraindications	Pregnancy, lactation, Kashin-Beck bone disease
Interactions	Anticoagulant/antiplatelet drugs, thyroid hormone replacement, immunosuppressants
Potential adverse effects	Diarrhea, headache, sore throat

Another related option that has become very popular recently is Himalayan shilajit extract. Shilajit is a mineral-rich resin with a rich history of traditional use in Ayurvedic medicine, where it is referred to as "rasayana," which means rejuvenator. It is formed from the decomposition of plant and microbial matter and contains 60–85 percent humic substances, fulvic acid, trace minerals, fatty acids, sterols, and phenolic lipids. The primary active compounds in shilajit are considered dibenzo-α-pyrones and fulvic acid and their derivatives. Unpurified shilajit has a urine-like odor because of its benzoic acid and benzoate content, making it important to use only purified extracts. Shilajit also acts as a binder and chelator because it contains humic substances and fulvic acid.[83,84] It is considered an adaptogen, and preclinical research suggests it helps decrease stress and anxiety and may even have a place in the prevention of cognitive disorders.[85,86] Clinical research demonstrated that taking 500 mg of shilajit (PrimaVie, a purified and standardized shilajit extract with $\geq$ 50% fulvic acid and $\geq$ 10.3% dibenzo-α-pyrones (DBP) + DPB chromoproteins) per day can reduce fatigue and help maintain muscular strength by promoting favorable muscle and connective tissue adaptations.[87] This activity makes sense since fulvic acid is a strong antioxidant and anti-inflammatory. Another clinical study found that taking 250 mg of shilajit (PrimaVie) twice daily for ninety consecutive days significantly increased total and free testosterone and dehydroepiandrosterone in healthy males aged 45 to 55.[88] Since low testosterone is seen in aging men and is associated with loss of muscle mass, fatigue, and increased body fat, shilajit has great potential to improve the quality of life among older men. Shilajit doesn't just aid men's health, though. It also has benefits for women. One randomized controlled clinical study evaluated the effects of shilajit supplementation (PrimaVie) on reducing postmenopausal bone loss.[89] Sixty postmenopausal women with osteopenia were randomized to receive placebo, 250 mg shilajit, or 500 mg of shilajit daily for forty-eight weeks. Daily supplementation resulted in improved bone mineral density and reduced inflammatory and oxidative markers, with the 500 mg group experiencing the greatest benefits. A whole host of benefits may be realized with shilajit since it combats aging related to mitochondrial dysfunction and works synergistically with CoQ10 to boost energy, preserve mitochondria, and reduce cellular aging. While many of its benefits are related to age-related conditions, young men and women report feeling better when they take it as well.

A quality purified shilajit supplement is imperative for benefits because a counterfeit or unpurified product may contain mycotoxins, heavy metals, or other potentially harmful compounds. A poor-quality supplement may also lack sufficient DBP, DBO chromoproteins, and fulvic acid to have effects. If shilajit is energizing to you, take it in the morning. If it makes you feel more relaxed, take it in the evening. Shilajit usually takes eight to twelve weeks to experience significant results and changes in your well-being.

SHILAJIT EXTRACT (Purified; ≥ 40% fulvic acid and ≥ 10% DBP + DPB chromoproteins)	
Typical dose	As instructed on the product label after a meal; 250–1,000 mg/day is commonly used, usually starting at the lower end and increasing the amount slowly
Cautions and contraindications	Pregnancy, lactation, and hemochromatosis
Interactions	Blood thinners, immunosuppressants, diabetic drugs, testosterone replacement
Potential adverse effects	Nausea, diarrhea, upset stomach, heartburn, headache, dizziness

Don't Ignore Lifestyle Adjustments!

Ignoring dietary sources of histamine is like using a small cup to bail water out of your histamine bathtub without first shutting off the histamine faucet. You don't have to modify your diet entirely, but you do need to make some positive adjustments to lower histamine levels. Sleep is an oft-ignored but vitally important factor in all aspects of your health. Rest well—feel well! Moreover, aiding your natural detoxification and elimination channels is essential for resolving symptoms of histamine intolerance and optimum health. Over time, you will feel better and improve your quality of life.

4

THE THREEFOLD APPROACH TO EFFECTIVELY MANAGING HISTAMINE INTOLERANCE: OPTIMIZE HISTAMINE METABOLISM

Beyond reducing the input of histamine into the body through dietary modifications, you need to support your body in metabolizing histamine. A DAO supplement is an obvious choice as it supplements your body's own production of this important histamine-metabolizing enzyme. DAO can be isolated from animals (e.g., pig kidneys); by germinating grains—pea (*Psium sativum*), grass pea (*Lathryus sativus*), or lentil (*Lens culinaris*); or from yeast (*Yarrowia lipolytica* PO1f). Their potency is measured in histamine-degrading units (HDUs). Both DAO deficiency and histamine intolerance can be managed with a DAO supplement as underlying causes are corrected. Normal values of DAO activity in people without histamine intolerance should be greater than 10 U/mL.[90] Anything lower than this is considered probable histamine intolerance.

Consider Taking a DAO Enzyme Supplement

DAO from grass pea was stable when exposed to a simulated gastrointestinal environment, except in the presence of alcohol (ethanol).[91] From this, we can conclude that DAO from plant sources should remain active in an intestinal environment as long as alcohol is not consumed. Evaluation of its efficacy to reduce symptoms of histamine intolerance was also performed in laboratory and *ex vivo* assays. What the researchers found was that plant-based DAO reduced colonic spasms caused by histamine.[92] Even more important, rectally administered plant-based DAO can be retained in the gut mucosa and remain active to metabolize and degrade histamine. Furthermore, a comparison of lyophilized pea DAO and pig DAO demonstrated that the pea-based DAO had the greatest histamine-degrading activity.[93] Contrarily, a review of DAO activity in ten commercially available dietary supplements showed that pig-based DAO supplements exhibited the greatest activity, with a plant-based supplement close behind.[94] Of those tested, DAOfood Plus (4.2 mg pig-based DAO, 40 mg quercetin, 20 mg vitamin C), DAOfood (4.2 mg pig-based DAO), and DAOfood Veg (4.2 mg pea shoots containing 0.3 mg DAO) were the most active, followed by DAOSIN (4.2 mg pig-based DAO, providing 0.3 mg DAO).

Yeast-based DAO Supplements

A simulated gastrointestinal model was also employed to determine the stability and effectiveness of DAO obtained from yeast and formulated with catalase as a sucrose-based tablet.[95] The tablet was introduced into the simulated intestinal conditions in the presence of food constituents and showed it degraded about thirty percent of histamine in ninety minutes. Stability was also confirmed in an environment similar to intestinal fluid. Altogether, the supplement showed sufficient histamine degradation to help people with histamine intolerance.

Pig Protein-based DAO Supplements

Conversely, DAO derived from pigs did not perform as well in a simulated gastrointestinal environment.[96] Much of the histamine reduction observed in this study was due to histamine adhering to the DAO capsule, not from increased DAO activity. Only a 12.1 percent reduction in histamine was attributed to the actual DAO in the capsule. The researchers concluded that pig-derived DAO does not adequately reduce histamine to manage histamine intolerance in humans sufficiently. Despite this, clinical research that will be shared below demonstrates meaningful reductions in histamine intolerance symptoms through supplementation with a pig-derived DAO enzyme.

Limited emerging research confirms the benefits of DAO supplementation for people with histamine intolerance. A small pilot clinical study involving fourteen people (thirteen adults and one child) with histamine intolerance and without food allergies (milk, egg, fish, shrimp, soy, nuts, and dried fruits), nickel allergies, celiac's, chronic hives, gastroesophageal reflux disease, gastric ulcer, and autoimmune conditions was performed.[97] The participants, who had previously experienced some relief by practicing a histamine-limiting diet, took a DAO supplement (DAOSIN—from pig kidneys providing 0.3 mg DAO; 10,000 HDUs) fifteen minutes before lunch and dinner for at least fourteen days. Participants were also asked to maintain or restart a low-histamine diet during the study. At the conclusion of the study, all but one participant reported relief of at least one digestive symptom after taking the DAO supplement.

Another open-label clinical study with twenty-eight participants diagnosed with histamine intolerance evaluated DAOSIN supplementation for four weeks and then followed participants for four weeks after stopping supplementation.[98] They took the DAO capsules before meals, up to three times daily, and were told not to alter their current diet or medications. All symptoms—digestive, cardiovascular, respiratory, and skin—of histamine intolerance dramatically improved while taking DAOSIN. Symptoms increased during the four-week follow-up period when DAOSIN was discontinued. This study suggests that DAO supplementation can improve symptoms of histamine intolerance without dietary modification, particularly if taken with each meal of the day.

As mentioned earlier, frequent migraines can be a symptom of histamine intolerance and DAO deficiency. A one-month randomized placebo-controlled clinical study including one hundred people with episodic migraines evaluated DAO supplementation as a solution.[99] Study participants in the intervention group took two DAOSIN capsules twenty minutes before each meal, whereas the placebo group took microcrystalline cellulose and gelatin capsules. Researchers observed a 22.5 percent reduction in the duration of migraine attacks— 1.4 hours on average—in the DAO supplement group. Only a small, nonsignificant reduction in migraine duration was observed in the control group. The DAO group also required fewer triptan migraine medications. The results of the study are promising and indicate that DAO supplementation may be helpful in reducing migraine duration.

Chronic spontaneous hives (urticaria) are driven by mast cells and usually involve the absence of clearly identifiable triggers. A randomized, double-blind, placebo-controlled clinical trial assessed the benefits of taking a DAO supplement in twenty-two people with chronic spontaneous hives incompletely controlled by first-line antihistamines and who were nonresponsive to a twenty-one-day histamine-free diet.[100] The participants were observed without treatment for fifteen days, followed by thirty days of taking DAOSIN (one capsule fifteen minutes before lunch and dinner), and then a fifteen-day washout period was observed before crossing over the placebo and intervention groups. A significant reduction in hives was noted among those with low DAO levels at the start of the trial, and a slight reduction in antihistamine use was observed among participants in the DAO group. Based on this, it can be concluded that hives among people with low DAO activity may be improved by DAO supplementation.

The available evidence suggests that people with histamine intolerance and related conditions who have deficient DAO levels or activity can benefit from supplemental DAO. A high-quality supplement with sufficient DAO activity is required to experience benefits. According to research, DAOfood Plus, DAOfood, and DAOfood Veg are high-quality supplements with excellent DAO activity. People without these deficiencies in levels or activity may not experience relief in symptoms.

DAO SUPPLEMENT (minimum 10,000 HDU)	
Typical dose	One (1) capsule 15 minutes before each meal; maximum of two (2) capsules three times daily before meals
Cautions and contraindications	Pregnancy, lactation

Interactions	None currently known, although it is possible that drugs that inhibit DAO activity in the body may interfere with supplements as well
Potential adverse effects	Nausea, headache, hives, lethargy, flu-like symptoms

Vital Nutrients for Healthy DAO Activity

Not surprisingly, many nutrients play a role in or are critical for healthy DAO activity. Vitamin B6, vitamin C, and copper are essential cofactors for DAO to function properly.[101,102,103] A clinical study confirmed that fatty acids and nutrients significantly influenced DAO activity in healthy women.[104] Specifically, intake of long-chain fatty acids, saturated fatty acids, and monounsaturated fatty acids, as well as phosphorus, calcium, zinc, magnesium, iron, and vitamin B12, were strongly correlated with serum DAO activity. Essentially, these nutrients activate the DAO enzyme, and deficiencies in any of them may contribute to decreased DAO activity. Other research concluded that serum DAO levels were influenced by a woman's menstrual cycle, with higher serum levels detected during the luteal phase.[105] Clinicians should be aware of this detail and determine the phase of the menstrual cycle in premenopausal women to avoid erroneous data from blood work. Given their importance as cofactors in stimulating DAO activity, it is important to supply the body with these nutrients when supplementing with DAO.

Vitamin B6

Also known as pyridoxine, vitamin B6 is an essential vitamin that helps maintain the health of your whole body. It is particularly important for immune and nervous system function. DAO activity is dependent on B6. Without sufficient levels of B6, DAO cannot be produced by your body successfully, nor can DAO metabolize histamine efficiently. Clinical research shows that taking 5 mg of pyridoxal-5'-phosphate for three to six months increases plasma-DAO activity but is not as pronounced in individuals who are deficient in B6 at the beginning of the trial.[106] Evidence from this study suggests that people with significant B6 deficiencies may require higher dosing or need to take it for longer to optimize levels for peak DAO activity. Other research showed that taking B6 is helpful for symptoms of histamine intolerance associated with wine drinking.[107] Drinking alcohol negatively affects B vitamins by reducing their effectiveness in the body and removing them from the body, so this finding is not surprising. Given its crucial role in DAO activity, B6 supplementation is important if you have histamine intolerance.

Vitamin C

While vitamin C is not known to prevent the release of histamine from cells, it is responsible for reducing histamine levels in your body. Levels of histamine in the blood are directly correlated with vitamin C levels. To illustrate this connection, we can look at studies correlating vitamin C with motion sickness. Seasickness is chiefly driven by elevated histamine levels in the brain, which is why most drugs used to treat seasickness are antihistamines. A double-blind placebo-controlled crossover study evaluated the effects of vitamin C in seventy volunteers who spent twenty minutes in a life raft exposed to rough waters to trigger seasickness.[108] Before being exposed to large waves in the life raft, volunteers were given 2,000 mg of vitamin C or a placebo on the first day of the experiment. The next day, the volunteers repeated the raft experience, with those who received vitamin C getting a placebo and the placebo group getting vitamin C. Elevated histamine levels were observed in both groups, but it was less pronounced in those who took vitamin C. Additionally, DAO levels increased more dramatically in the vitamin C groups. Seasickness symptoms were suppressed by vitamin C intake, with women and men under age twenty-seven receiving the most benefits. The findings of the research show that vitamin C intake is linked to improved histamine degradation and DAO activity.

Copper

Copper is a cofactor for several enzymes involved in energy production, neurotransmitter creation, neuropeptide activation, iron metabolism, and connective tissue synthesis. It also plays a role in the formation of new blood vessels, neurohormone balance, gene expression, immune function, and brain development. Another potential cause of low DAO activity is copper deficiency. Low copper levels have been linked to decreased DAO levels and activity in the blood.[109,110] Zinc prevents intestinal absorption of copper, so taking large amounts of zinc daily (likely over 100 mg) may contribute to deficiency. It is a good idea to check both zinc and copper levels and strive to maintain an ideal zinc-to-copper ratio of 8:1 (range 4:1 to 12:1).

Phosphorus

Phosphorus, an essential mineral, is a component of bones, teeth, DNA, and RNA. It is involved in the regulation of gene transcription, enzyme activation, maintenance of a healthy pH in extracellular fluid, and energy storage inside cells. As mentioned earlier, clinical research linked the dietary intake of phosphorus with healthy DAO activity. Strive to include foods rich in phosphorus, such as turkey, beef, chicken, cashews, rice, and eggs, in your diet.

Calcium

Known primarily for its essential role in bone health—although bone health depends more on its metabolism and the utilization of vitamin D, vitamin K, and magnesium than its intake—calcium is the most abundant mineral in the body. It makes up much of the structure of the bones and teeth but also aids cardiovascular function, nerve transmission, and hormone secretion. As a highly positively charged ion, calcium regulates the function of all cell types, making controlling calcium transport and its intracellular homeostasis crucial for biological function. DAO shows maximal activity when in the presence of calcium ions.[111] Calcium is also believed to release histamine from brain tissues, thus liberating it for metabolism and degradation and decreasing tissue burden in the body. So, calcium helps your body make more DAO and improves its activity.

Zinc

Zinc is involved in many aspects of cellular metabolism and essential to the activity of hundreds of enzymes. It plays a role in protein and DNA synthesis, cell signaling and division, immune function, and wound healing. Zinc inhibits the release of histamine by regulating both mast cells and basophils.[112] Its consumption is associated with improved DAO activity. Depletion of this crucial mineral leads to higher histamine levels in the body.

Magnesium

Magnesium has multiple functions in the human body, including energy production, muscle contraction, muscle function, and cardiovascular health. It acts as a cofactor for more than three hundred enzymatic reactions in the body. It has such an impact on human health that its deficiency has been associated with a wide range of diseases, such as cardiovascular disease and nervous system disorders. Magnesium is an important cofactor in the production of DAO, and its deficiency may lead to excess histamine levels. Moreover, a shortage of magnesium in the body increases histidine decarboxylase activity, which is the enzyme that makes histamine from histidine. An animal study found that histamine levels rapidly increased in magnesium-deficient rats.[113] Magnesium helps control histamine levels in two ways: by supporting the enzyme that breaks it down and by decreasing the enzyme that creates it.

Iron

Iron is an essential component of hemoglobin—a red blood cell protein that carries oxygen from the lungs to other tissues. Iron supports muscle metabolism, healthy connective tissue, cell functioning, and the creation of some hormones. Women who experience heavy bleeding during menstruation should have their iron and ferritin levels checked because they are more likely to have insufficient or deficient levels of iron. Iron deficiency primes mast cells and increases histamine release.[114] Mast cell activation can be limited by the addition of iron-containing proteins (transferrin, lactoferrin) or iron-loaded whey protein beta-lactoglobulin.[115] Dietary iron is correlated with DAO activity.

Vitamin B12

Vitamin B12 is required for healthy nervous system function, red blood cell formation, and DNA synthesis. It is a cofactor for methionine synthase and L-methylmalonyl-CoA mutase. Methionine synthase is essential to catalyze the conversion of homocysteine to methionine, which the body uses to form S-adenosylmethionine (SAMe). SAMe is a methyl donor for nearly one hundred substrates, including DNA, RNA, proteins, and lipids, making it vital for gene expression and epigenetic modification. Histamine metabolism is accelerated when sufficient SAMe is present in the body by supporting methylation. Sluggish methylation means fewer methyl groups to bind to a receptor site on a substance like histamine. When this occurs, histamine builds up in the body, causing an overload. Methylcobalamin and 5-deoxyadenosylcobalamin are metabolically active forms of vitamin B12. People with poor methylation (e.g., MTHFR mutations) should take a methylated form of B12. Nonmethylated forms, like hydroxocobalamin and cyanocobalamin, only become active after they are methylated in the body and converted to the bioactive forms. Not surprisingly, B12 plays a crucial role in your body's production of DAO, and without optimal levels, histamine can build up in the body quickly and trigger symptoms of histamine intolerance.

Multinutrient with Methylated B Vitamins and Chelated/ Complexed Minerals

A good multinutrient with methylated B vitamins and chelated or complexed minerals is a great place to start to ensure you are getting the cofactors to produce DAO and maintain its activity. Vitamin and nutrient levels should be evaluated to determine any deficiencies or subclinical deficiencies of these nutrients. If less than optimal levels are identified, higher levels of the deficient nutrient should be taken as recommended below.

VITAMIN B6 (pyridoxal-5'-phosphate; preferably as a B-complex)	
Typical dose	15–50 mg/day
Cautions and contraindications	Prior to surgery (especially angioplasty or bariatric surgery)
Interactions	High blood pressure drugs, amiodarone, barbiturates, antiseizure meds, cycloserine
Potential adverse effects	Very well tolerated, occasionally stomachache, headache, heartburn, nausea, vomiting, loss of appetite, and sleepiness are experienced
VITAMIN C (from camu camu or as ascorbyl palmitate) + BIOFLAVONOIDS	
Typical dose	1,000 mg, two or three times daily
Cautions and contraindications	Kidney stones, glucose-6-phosphate dehydrogenase (G6PD) deficiency
Interactions	Estrogen, antitumor antibiotics, warfarin, antipsychotics (fluphenazine), indinavir, aluminum-containing meds/products (increases absorption of aluminum)
Potential adverse effects	Very well tolerated, occasionally abdominal cramps, heartburn, esophagitis, diarrhea, nausea, vomiting, headache, and kidney stones (in individuals prone to them)
COPPER	
Typical dose	Generally not recommended as a supplement unless deficiency or suboptimal zinc-to-copper ratio is confirmed
Cautions and contraindications	Idiopathic copper toxicosis, Wilson disease
Interactions	Penicillamine (decreases copper absorption); iron, vitamin C, and zinc
Potential adverse effects	Well tolerated, occasionally stomachache, nausea, vomiting, diarrhea, headache, dizziness, weakness, and a metallic taste in the mouth

PHOSPHORUS	
Typical dose	From food sources, supplementation is usually not necessary
Cautions and contraindications	Chronic kidney disease
Interactions	Aspirin, digoxin, high blood pressure drugs, and diuretics; vitamin D and calcium
Potential adverse effects	Nausea, vomiting, diarrhea, stomachache or upset stomach, increased thirst, pain (muscle, joint, and bone)

CALCIUM (as malate)	
Typical dose	500 mg/day
Cautions and contraindications	Kidney dysfunction, sarcoidosis, and individuals with a higher risk of stroke
Interactions	Ceftriaxone, bisphosphonates, calcipotriene, digoxin, diltiazem, levothyroxine, lithium, quinolone antibiotics, tetracycline antibiotics, raltegravir, sotalol, thiazide diuretics, verapamil, and aluminum-containing meds/products (increases absorption of aluminum); iron, lycopene, magnesium, vitamin D, and zinc
Potential adverse effects	Very well tolerated, belching, constipation or diarrhea, flatulence, and stomachache

ZINC (as bisglycinate chelate)	
Typical dose	15 mg/day; as directed by a qualified health professional for deficiency
Cautions and contraindications	Chronic kidney disease
Interactions	Cephalexin, cisplatin, integrase inhibitors, penicillamine, quinolone antibiotics, tetracycline antibiotics, and ritonavir; beta-carotene, calcium, chromium, copper, folic

	acid, iron, magnesium, manganese, riboflavin, vitamin A, and vitamin D
Potential adverse effects	Well tolerated, occasionally abdominal cramps, diarrhea, nausea, vomiting, and a metallic taste in the mouth

MAGNESIUM (Complex with low/no citrate; or as bisglycinate chelate)

Typical dose	500 mg/day
Cautions and contraindications	Pregnancy, bleeding disorders, heart block, kidney dysfunction, myasthenia gravis
Interactions	Levodopa/carbidopa, aminoglycoside antibiotics, quinolone antibiotics, tetracycline antibiotics, antacids, bisphosphonates, calcium channel blockers, digoxin, ketamine, potassium-sparing diuretics, muscle relaxers, and sulfonylureas; herbs with antiplatelet or anticoagulant activity, boron, calcium, vitamin D, and zinc
Potential adverse effects	Very well tolerated, occasionally digestive upset, nausea, or vomiting

IRON (as ferrous bisglycinate)

Typical dose	Females: 18 mg/day during menstruation or 25 mg elemental iron from chelated iron every other day with deficiency; Males: only if deficiency or insufficiency is confirmed
Cautions and contraindications	Type 2 diabetes, hemoglobin diseases, hereditary hemorrhagic telangiectasia, and premature infants
Interactions	Bisphosphonates, dolutegravir, integrase inhibitors, levodopa, methyldopa, levothyroxine, mycophenolate mofetil, penicillamine, quinolone antibiotics, and tetracycline antibiotics; beta-carotene, calcium, vitamin A, vitamin C, and zinc
Potential adverse effects	Very well tolerated, occasionally abdominal pain, constipation, diarrhea, digestive upset, nausea, and vomiting

VITAMIN B12 (as methylcobalamin with L-methylfolate)	
Typical dose	500–2,000 mcg methylcobalamin + 1–15 mg L-methylfolate
Cautions and contraindications	Prior to surgery (especially) and cobalt or cobalamin hypersensitivity
Interactions	Colchicine, proton pump inhibitors, and metformin; potassium and vitamin C
Potential adverse effects	Very well tolerated, occasionally nausea, vomiting, diarrhea, headache, tingling sensation in hands or feet, and fatigue

Probiotics

Since DAO activity is primarily regulated in the gut, it makes complete sense that an imbalance in the microflora within the gut can contribute to histamine intolerance. This is particularly true when you consider that some gut bacteria are histamine secreters, which can result in a greater abundance of histamine in the body. The key is to have a balance of histamine degraders—*Escherichia coli* (H.1, H.9, and H.14), *Clostridium perfringens* isolates (B.1, B.2, and B.3), and *Klebsiella pneumoniae* (I.2)—and secreters that allows your body to efficiently control histamine levels.[116] These findings are interesting and suggest that specific strains within a species of bacteria are likely to have different effects on histamine in the body. It may be surprising to see these bacteria as histamine degraders since they are more commonly considered pathogenic and associated with human infections. However, nonpathogenic strains that are advantageous in the gut and provide health benefits also exist.

Indeed, mounting evidence supports that histamine intolerance begins in the gut.[117] Altered gut microbiome composition contributes to mucosal inflammation, a condition that impairs DAO activity.[118] Further supporting a gut origin of histamine intolerance, individuals with histamine intolerance have a higher prevalence of dysbiosis. A study compared the gut microbiome of healthy individuals with those diagnosed with histamine intolerance. What the researchers found was that people with histamine intolerance had a significantly lower proportion of *Prevotellaceae, Ruminococcus, Faecalibacterium,* and *Faecalibacterium prausnitzii,* which are bacteria important for gut health. They also had a significantly higher abundance of histamine-secreting bacteria such as *Staphylococcus, Proteus, Enterobacteriaceae, Clostridium perfringens* (pathogenic), and *Enterococcus faecalis.*[119] Overall health absolutely follows gut health, and gut health is largely controlled by the diversity and abundance of microbes in the gut.

Based on limited research, commercially available probiotic strains that may benefit histamine intolerance include *Lactobacillus rhamnosus, Bifidobacterium infantis, Bifidobacterium longum, Lactobacillus plantarum,* and possibly *Lactobacillus reuteri.* Strains tested in laboratory research include *Lactobacillus plantarum* D-1033 and *Lactobacillus rhamnosus* GG.[120] Specifically, these strains suppressed genes related to IgE-mediated allergies and histamine H4 receptors, and strongly influenced genes related to mast cell activity and inflammatory control when used as part of a multistrain probiotic. *Lactobacillus plantarum* D-103 displayed high histamine-degrading activity in preclinical research.[121] An animal model of nasal allergies found that Lac-B (a mixture of freeze-dried *Bifidobacterium infantis* and *Bifidobacterium longum*) demonstrated that Lac-B suppresses histamine H1 receptors and histidine decarboxylase mRNA expression, therefore reducing overall histamine levels.[122] In other words, this probiotic interferes with histamine signaling and may be able to reduce histamine intolerance and related symptoms. *Lactobacillus reuteri* 6475 contains a complete chromosomal histidine decarboxylase gene cluster, which gives it the capacity to convert histidine to histamine.[123] While this may seem like a bad thing, *L. reuteri*–produced histamine actually has an anti-inflammatory effect on the gut, activating anti-inflammatory H2 receptors and suppressing pro-inflammatory H1 receptors.[124] Additionally, it is important for folate metabolism, an important function to reduce excessive histamine production. Based on this, these strains should be prioritized in your probiotic supplement, while *Lactobacillus bulgaricus*, *Lactobacillus saerimneri*, and *Lactobacillus casei* should be strictly limited or avoided when addressing histamine intolerance due to their known histamine-secreting properties.

PROBIOTIC (Multistrain)	
Typical dose	At least 10 billion CFUs/AFUs containing eight or more strains, with evening meal
Cautions and contraindications	None currently known
Interactions	Antibiotics and antifungals
Potential adverse effects	Very well tolerated, occasionally mild digestive discomfort

MTHFR Mutations and Methylation Defects

For those with MTHFR mutations, it is possible that you have a methylation defect, but not always. Histamine levels are directly correlated with your methylation function since methylation is used to control the amount of histamine inside cells. Whole blood histamine and plasma methylation levels are the best way to determine your current methylation status. The presence of an MTFHR mutation, even homozygous mutations, does not always mean you have a methylation defect, so blood testing is important to determine your status. If whole blood histamine is low, you are overmethylated, and if whole blood histamine levels are high, you are undermethylated. You may also bounce back and forth between under and overmethylation. Note that it takes at least three or four months to correct methylation defects, and the nutrients used to correct the defect must be taken indefinitely since they do not fix the underlying genetic mutation.

At its simplest, methylation and demethylation is the transfer of methyl groups—simple structures with one carbon and three hydrogen molecules (CH_3)—from one molecule to another. It biochemically modifies DNA and other molecules, which may be retained in future cells as cells divide. Functional products in the body, like proteins, enzymes, and hormones, rely on methylation to perform optimally. Methylation is critical for gene expression, DNA replication, and DNA repair, all of which require sufficient folate. This process is also necessary for the creation of the primary neurotransmitters and catecholamines serotonin, melatonin, dopamine, norepinephrine, and epinephrine. Methylation is one of the liver's six main pathways for detoxification and the generation of glutathione, your body's master antioxidant. It is also one way the body detoxifies and eliminates sex hormones not necessary for immediate use. When a section of DNA is methylated, it prevents RNA polymerases from reading it and controls gene expression—represses (promoter methylation) or activates (gene body) gene expression depending on where methylation occurs in the DNA sequence. Demethylation does the opposite, removing a methyl group and typically activating the gene. Think of this process as a copy machine. Methylated DNA is like placing a black sheet over part of the paper you want to copy. The black sheet will obviously prevent copying that part of the document. Demethylation removes the black sheet from the document so that that section can be read and actively used again. Methylation is all about balance because too much methylation can be as problematic as too little. You don't want to undermethylate or overmethylate (also called hypermethylation). You want to find the sweet spot of optimal methylation. A person who can methylate and demethylate efficiently will be healthier because their cells are more adaptable to the constantly changing environment in the body.

Some signs or symptoms of overmethylation include anxiety, depression, sleep troubles, hyperactivity, food sensitivities or allergies, absence of seasonal allergies, tendency to be overweight, nervous legs, pacing, rapid speech, excessive body hair, low libido, overly fervent religious state, dry eyes or mouth, poor motivation, tinnitus, highly artistic, musically inclined, copper overload, estrogen and antihistamine intolerance, high serotonin levels, adverse reactions to SSRI antidepressants or SAMe, and improvement with benzodiazepines. Contrastingly, undermethylation is associated with perfectionism, chronic depression, compulsive, ritualistic behaviors, seasonal allergies, phobias, addictive tendencies, strong willed, self-motivated (especially during school years), highly competitive, social isolation, calm disposition but inwardly very tense, frequent headaches, slender, inflexible food choices, terse speech, sparse body hair, low serotonin, strong libido, adverse reaction to benzodiazepines and folic acid, and improvement with SSRI antidepressants and antihistamines.

Beyond the elimination of histamine-associated foods mentioned earlier, those with methylation defects may see improvement through further dietary modification. Overmethylators should consume moderate amounts of protein to avoid the overproduction of serotonin and increase plant-based foods, particularly those rich in folate (e.g., beans, asparagus, spinach, leafy greens, avocados). The amino acid precursors to the production of glutathione—cysteine, glycine, and glutamate—are particularly important. Alcohol should be avoided since it can increase the risk of overmethylation. Copper-to-zinc ratio should be assessed because overmethylators frequently have a high copper-to-zinc ratio, which means copper supplements could make things worse, and zinc supplements may improve symptoms. Avoid foods enriched with copper.

Undermethylators will often thrive on a high-protein, animal-based diet because animal proteins are more similar to human proteins, making them more bioavailable. This includes supporting methylation cycle enzymes involved in the creation of SAMe, homocysteine, and creatine. Predominantly plant-based diets do not provide all of the nutrients required for optimal methylation and glutathione synthesis regardless of methylation status but are particularly detrimental to undermethylators. Emphasize whole, fresh, unprocessed foods. Fresh grass-fed and grass-finished beef, wild-caught fish, and grass-fed organ meats are high in key amino acids—cysteine, glycine, and glutamine—to support glutathione synthesis. Limit or eliminate grains and replace them with nuts and seeds (except seed oils), fruit (especially berries), free-range eggs, quality fats (coconut, ghee, grass-fed butter, and olive oil), and moderate amounts of some vegetables. At the same time, foods rich in folate can increase your reuptake of serotonin in the brain, effectively decreasing serotonin concentrations. Look for nutritional imbalances such as protein, calcium, magnesium, and vitamin B6. Avoid extreme detox or cleansing protocols that can deplete your body of vital nutrients. Molecules obtained by diet are used by the body to promote the expression of our genes, making choosing foods for our bio-individuality critical. There is no one-size-fits-all approach to nutrition!

UNDERMETHYLATORS— METHYLFOLATE + METHYLCOBALAMIN	
Typical dose	500–2,000 mcg sublingual methylcobalamin + 1–15 mg L-methylfolate
Cautions and contraindications	Prior to surgery (especially) and cobalt or cobalamin hypersensitivity
Interactions	Colchicine, proton pump inhibitors, and metformin; potassium and vitamin C
Potential adverse effects	Very well tolerated, occasionally nausea, vomiting, diarrhea, headache, tingling sensation in hands or feet, and fatigue

Serine is generally considered a nonessential amino acid involved in nucleotide and lipid metabolism and physiological growth. It is very important to maintain metabolic homeostasis and health during stressful situations or pathological states. It can be conditionally essential because serine levels in the body are usually insufficient during pathological states or infections. Serine is also involved in glutathione balance and decreases overmethylation, according to preclinical models.[125] Higher glutathione concentrations protect against cellular and tissue damage and ease disease progression.

OVERMETHYLATORS— GLUTATHIONE + SERINE	
Typical dose	*Glutathione*: 100 mg S-Acetyl L-Glutathione daily with a meal *Serine*: 2,000 mg L-serine per day

Cautions and contraindications	Glutathione: Pregnancy and lactation Serine: Pregnancy, lactation, and kidney disease
Interactions	Glutathione: None currently known Serine: None currently known
Potential adverse effects	Glutathione: Very well tolerated, rarely abdominal cramping and bloating Serine: Very well tolerated, occasionally abdominal pain, bloating, nausea, upset stomach, and loss of appetite

Promoting Histamine Balance

Aiding your body's efforts to metabolize histamine and promote histamine balance so your body gets the benefits of histamine without the adverse effects is a vital part of your histamine intolerance improvement plan. Providing nutrients that support DAO activity, supplementing your DAO enzyme levels, improving gut microbiome diversity, and addressing methylation defects are fundamental steps to relief. Be patient and consistent for best results.

5

THE THREEFOLD APPROACH TO EFFECTIVELY MANAGING HISTAMINE INTOLERANCE: STABILIZE DEGRANULATING CELLS

The next step in addressing histamine intolerance is to reduce histamine release, predominantly by stabilizing degranulating cells. One caution with this step is to use only one mast cell stabilizer at a time. While too much histamine and inflammation are harmful, too little is also bad, suppressing functions like muscle repair.

Quercetin

First on the list is quercetin, which is a plant flavonoid in the polyphenol class and an antioxidant found in many fruits, vegetables, and grains. The great thing about quercetin is that it has multiple biological activities, among which mast cell stabilizing, inhibiting pro-inflammatory cytokine release, and gastrointestinal protective activity are among the most relevant to histamine intolerance.[126,127,128] Mast cell stabilizers block the release of histamine and related mediators by stabilizing the cell's membrane. In addition, quercetin plays an important role in regulating gut permeability and the health of the gut microbiome.[129] Lastly, quercetin improves the Th1/Th2 balance and suppresses antigen-specific IgE antibody formation, making it effective for allergic symptoms like those experienced by people with histamine intolerance.[130] Thus, quercetin works to reduce histamine release from mast cells, including intestinal cells, serving as a natural antihistamine and reducing symptoms of histamine intolerance.

QUERCETIN	
Typical dose	400–500 mg quercetin, two to three times daily with a meal; or 250 mg quercetin LipoMicel Matrix, two to three times daily
Cautions and contraindications	Pregnancy, lactation, bleeding disorders, and kidney disorders
Interactions	Blood-pressure-lowering drugs, blood-thinning drugs, quinolone antibiotics, immunosuppressant drugs
Potential adverse effects	Headache and tingling of extremities

Bioflavonoid Complex

Other bioflavonoids that could be considered are fisetin, kaempferol, myricetin, luteolin, and rutin. These flavonoids also reduce the release of histamine and pro-inflammatory mediators from mast cells and basophils.[131,132] Flavonoids are known to directly influence the activation and maturation of immune cells and regulate cytokine generation, immune cell secretion, and cellular communication. Their multiple mechanisms and profound effects on immune cells and function make them promising solutions for a variety of allergic inflammatory conditions involving excessive mast cell activation, including histamine intolerance.

BIOFLAVONOID COMPLEX	
Typical dose	As instructed on the product label
Cautions and contraindications	Pregnancy, lactation, bleeding disorders, and liver or kidney disease
Interactions	Blood-pressure-lowering drugs, blood-thinning drugs, quinolone antibiotics, immunosuppressant drugs

Potential adverse effects	Headache, dizziness, nervousness, skin redness or itching, heavy feeling in legs or feet, irregular heartbeat, and blurred vision

Berberine

A bioactive alkaloid extracted from several plants, most commonly Indian barberry, berberine has been used in traditional Chinese medicine for a host of ailments, including high blood sugar, heart conditions, high cholesterol, and for weight loss. Cellular and animal models demonstrate that berberine significantly inhibits IgE-mediated mast cell degranulation and their release of histamine, β-hexosaminidase, and pro-inflammatory mediators.[133] Additionally, it suppressed mechanisms involved in allergic reactions, including anaphylactic reactions. The results of the research suggest that berberine can reduce mast cell activation and suppress allergic reactions. Another study found that berberine effectively regulates pathways involved in histidine and nicotinamide metabolism.[134] In relation to histamine intolerance, the findings show that berberine may help the body better metabolize histidine (the amino acid precursor to histamine), which may improve symptoms of histamine intolerance. Moreover, its effects on nicotinamide metabolism may reduce excess histamine and serotonin levels because surplus nicotinamide in the body disrupts monoamine-neurotransmitter metabolism and interferes with methylation.[135] Make sure your berberine comes from Indian barberry plant roots and not bark. The bark is higher in salicylates, and some people have reported that supplements from the bark trigger a skin reaction, particularly those sensitive to salicylates.

BERBERINE	
Typical dose	400–600 mg, two to three times daily, with meals
Cautions and contraindications	Pregnancy, lactation
Interactions	Cyclosporine, diabetes drugs, metformin, blood-thinning drugs, blood-pressure-

	lowering drugs, CNS depressant drugs, benzodiazepines, statins, barbiturates, dextromethorphan, immunosuppressive meds
Potential adverse effects	Generally well tolerated orally, abdominal pain or distension, diarrhea, constipation, flatulence, nausea, vomiting

Stinging Nettle

Urtica is a genus of flower plants, many of which have stinging hairs that go by the name nettles. Stinging nettle (*Urtica dioica*) has a centuries-long history of use for muscle and joint pain, gout, anemia, and eczema, and is the most common nettle used for allergies. Stinging nettle contains quercetin, which may be its active constituent. Preclinical research found that stinging nettle blocks histamine H1 receptors and inhibits mast cell tryptase, which prevents mast cells from degranulating and releasing histamine and pro-inflammatory molecules.[136] It also reduces inflammation by suppressing prostaglandin production via multiple mechanisms.[137] Clinical research found that taking 150 mg of stinging nettle reduced symptoms of allergic rhinitis, but the placebo group also experienced relief, casting doubt on its clinical efficacy.[138] Nevertheless, many people find relief from histamine-related symptoms when using stinging nettle, particularly when it is used as part of an herbal complex.

STINGING NETTLE	
Typical dose	150–750 mg per day
Cautions and contraindications	Pregnancy, lactation
Interactions	Antidiabetic drugs, diuretics, warfarin, lithium
Potential adverse effects	Well tolerated, constipation and diarrhea

Butterbur

Probably best known for its relief of migraines— the American Headache Society gave the herb a level A recommendation and declared it effective in preventing migraine headaches[139]—butterbur (*Petasites hybridus*) is also used for seasonal allergies and asthma. It contains petasins and a compound called petatewalide B, which suppresses the activation of ß-hexosaminidase mast cells.[140] Petatewalide B also reduces inflammation by inhibiting nitric oxide synthase. Researchers consider butterbur an antiallergic remedy because of its dual role in blocking leukotriene creation (leukotrienes play pivotal roles in inflammation and allergies) and the binding of histamine to H1-receptors (antihistamine).[141,142] People experiencing allergic rhinitis reported significant relief of nasal symptoms when taking two tablets of butterbur (standardized to 8 mg of petasins per tablet) three times daily after only five days of use.[143] Remarkably, histamine levels were reduced from 153.7 to 53.0 pg/mL and leukotrienes from 137.0 to 70.1 pg/mL during the intervention period. Another randomized crossover clinical study found that taking 25 mg of butterbur, twice daily, for one week reduced symptoms of allergic asthma when used in combination with inhaled corticosteroids.[144] Significant reductions in inflammation and eosinophil counts were noted during the study period. Based on anecdotal reports of histamine intolerance relief by taking butterbur extract, researchers investigated the effects of a standardized butterbur extract on DAO and HNMT activity and the organic cation transporter 3 (OCT3; a contributor to the transport of histamine through cells).[145] The findings showed that butterbur does not influence DAO or HNMT activity. Instead, it suppresses OCT, therefore limiting cellular transport of histamine. These studies prove that butterbur is fast-acting and symptomatic relief from histamine-related conditions, which should be experienced within one week of use.

BUTTERBUR EXTRACT (pyrrolizidine alkaloid-free)	
Typical dose	50 mg, two to three times daily
Cautions and contraindications	Pregnancy, lactation, liver disease (many practitioners recommend monitoring liver

	enzymes while taking butterbur, even in healthy individuals)
Interactions	Anticholinergic drugs
Potential adverse effects	Generally well tolerated, upset stomach, belching, diarrhea, headache, itchy eyes, general itching, rash, drowsiness, fatigue

Ginger

Preclinical research suggests that ginger extract also acts as a histamine blocker and may help reduce histamine-related gut inflammation. This makes sense because antihistamines are one class of drugs used to reduce nausea and vomiting since nausea and motion sickness are caused by histamine. Nonsteroidal anti-inflammatory drugs are known to be hard on the stomach and may cause stomach ulcers partly by increasing intestinal peroxides, inflammation, and histamine levels. An animal study found that ingestion of ginger extract protected against oxidative damage, intestinal inflammation, and excessive histamine release.[146] As an added benefit, ginger supports healthy immune function. A mouse model of allergic rhinitis found that adding ginger powder to food reduced IgE levels and mast cell activity, and one of its active compounds, 6-gingerol, suppressed the activation of T lymphocytes, which are immune cells that play a critical role in allergy symptoms.[147] With a wide safety tolerance and multiple effects, ginger extract is worth exploring for the relief of histamine intolerance symptoms.

GINGER	
Typical dose	500 mg, two to three times daily; or 100–150 mg of ginger extract standardized to minimum 20% gingeroids ($\geq$ 40% is better), once daily
Cautions and contraindications	Pregnancy, bleeding conditions, heart conditions, prior to surgery
Interactions	Anticoagulant and antiplatelet meds, antidiabetic drugs, losartan, nifedipine, phenprocoumon, warfarin; anticoagulant and

	antiplatelet supplements, supplements that affect blood sugar levels
Potential adverse effects	Well tolerated up to 5 grams daily, abdominal discomfort, diarrhea, belching, heartburn

Coenzyme Q10

Don't overlook supporting mitochondrial function as part of your strategy. Given their diverse roles and functions in the body and direct connection to mast cell degranulation, a supplement to support their function is valuable. One of the leading supplements to support mitochondrial function is coenzyme Q10 (CoQ10). Naturally produced by the body, CoQ10 is a powerful antioxidant and a key component of mitochondrial function. It is linked to pathways that not only regulate mitochondrial function but also metabolic pathways in other parts of the cell, giving it the ability to affect metabolic pathways outside the mitochondria as well.[148] Preclinical models show that CoQ10 supplementation activates nuclear factor erythroid 2-related factor 2 (NRF2), which is a pathway that regulates cellular defenses against toxic and oxidative insults.[149] Activation of NRF2 improves cellular resistance to allergic inflammatory responses. Moreover, CoQ10 served to moderate allergic factors such as histamine and IgE. CoQ10 is particularly important to supplement if you take a statin because statins are known to deplete this vital nutrient.[150] While mostly an indirect effect, CoQ10, when taken in sufficient doses, may increase cellular resilience and metabolism.

COQ10 (Ubiquinol)	
Typical dose	150 mg, one to four times daily
Cautions and contraindications	Pregnancy, lactation
Interactions	Warfarin, alkylating chemotherapy agents
Potential adverse effects	Very well tolerated, stomach upset, appetite suppression, diarrhea, heartburn, nausea, vomiting

Urolithin A

Another possible way to support healthy mitochondrial function, specifically by stimulating mitophagy, is by supplementing with urolithin A. Urolithin A is a natural compound produced by gut bacteria through the metabolism of ingested ellagitannins and ellagic acid (complex polyphenols found abundantly in pomegranate, berries, and nuts). High levels of ellagic acid or ellagitannins can be found in pomegranates, strawberries, blackberries, camu camu, walnuts, chestnuts, pistachios, and pecans. The conversion of ellagitannins and ellagic acid to urolithin A is much higher in individuals who have a diverse gut microbiome with higher levels of Firmicutes to Bacteroides, suggesting a healthy gut may be necessary to get this key metabolite without supplementation.[151] Multiple preclinical studies suggest that urolithin A protects against aging (prolongs lifespan) and age-related conditions involving muscles, the brain, joints, and other organs.[152] One of the mechanisms by which it protects against these conditions is by activating mitophagy.[153] Mitochondrial dysfunction is a recognized hallmark of aging. Clinical research shows that ingesting 500 or 1,000 mg of urolithin A improves the expression of mitochondrial genes in skeletal muscle, resulting in enhanced muscular endurance and decreased inflammatory markers in older adults.[154] While your gut microbiome can and does manufacture this important metabolite, supplementing with it may increase its beneficial effects, and clinical research confirms it markedly increases urolithin A levels in the blood compared to ingesting precursors to its production, like pomegranate juice.[155] In other words, you must have the right bacteria in your gut to convert precursors from foods into beneficial urolithin A. Production is also dependent upon health status and age, meaning the older you get, the less urolithin A you are likely to produce. Limited emerging research indicates that supplemental urolithin A can protect against histamine-induced damage and cell death.[156] At the very least, the available evidence suggests that urolithin A can enhance healthspan, protect against age-related conditions, preserve mitochondrial function and cellular metabolism by sparking mitophagy, and shield against histamine-related damage and symptoms.

UROLITHIN A (Liposomal)[157]	
Typical dose	500–1,500 mg/day
Cautions and contraindications	None currently known
Interactions	None currently known
Potential adverse effects	Very well tolerated, nausea, diarrhea

Essential Oils

Essential oils are ideal remedies for a variety of conditions because of their potency, privileged access to tissues (a small molecular weight and size means they can get to tissues that are traditionally challenging to access), and intrinsic polypharmacology (multiple constituents that have additive, synergistic, and antagonistic effects). Some essential oils can stabilize mast cells and decrease their degranulation. One of the most popular essential oils is lavender (*Lavandula angustifolia*), and it is affectionately called the "Swiss army knife" of essential oils because of its many uses. Preclinical research shows that lavender can stabilize mast cells and reduce their release of allergy-causing chemicals.[158,159] German chamomile (*Matricaria recutita*) essential oil inhibits mast cell degranulation, which reduces the release of histamine.[160] Himalayan cedarwood (*Cedrus deodara*) essential oil, which is very similar in composition to Atlas cedarwood (*Cedrus atlantica*) essential oil, balances mast cell activity and suppresses their release of pro-inflammatory leukotrienes.[161] Copaiba (*Copaifera* spp.) essential oil contains the highest amounts of beta-caryophyllene among currently known essential oils. This sesquiterpene and irregular cannabinoid has been shown to suppress the release of histamine and pro-inflammatory mediators by mast cells.[162] Additionally, it can bind to endocannabinoid type 2 receptors found throughout the body to support immune health and a healthy inflammatory response. Anecdotally, people report that lemon (*Citrus limon*), peppermint (*Mentha piperita*), and ginger (*Zingiber officinale*) essential oils are also helpful in reducing allergies. Based on the above research and user reports, one could take a capsule filled with two drops each of lavender, German chamomile, and copaiba, and one drop each of lemon and peppermint twice daily.

EO CAPSULE (2 drops: lavender, German chamomile, and copaiba, and 1 drop: lemon and peppermint)	
Typical dose	Twice daily
Cautions and contraindications	Pregnancy, lactation, ventricular fibrillation, iron deficiency, iron-deficiency anemia, GERD
Interactions	Cyclosporine, 5-fluorouracil, antibiotics, antifungals, aspirin, blood pressure-lowering drugs, anticholinergics and cholinergics
Potential adverse effects	Well tolerated, burp back, heartburn

Finding Relief through Stabilizing Degranulating Cells

You may not need to resort to antihistamines. There are many natural solutions to stabilize mast cells and reduce their degranulation and release of histamine and pro-inflammatory mediators. This is one of the best things you can do for histamine intolerance. Such natural solutions have different potencies and efficacies, so it may take trying one for a while and then switching to another if you don't get the relief you desire. CoQ10 and urolithin A can be used in combination with one of the aforementioned mast cell stabilizers since they work by different mechanisms and act complementary. You may find great relief through these natural products with good safety profiles.

6

REGAIN A HIGH QUALITY OF LIFE AND SAY GOODBYE TO HISTAMINE INTOLERANCE

Living with the symptoms of histamine intolerance is tricky because the symptoms are often confused with other conditions, such as seasonal allergies. Unfortunately, many practitioners are not familiar with histamine intolerance to even consider diagnosing it. To make matters worse, histamine levels and DAO activity are unlikely to be tested unless your practitioner is familiar with histamine intolerance and does so on a hunch or you request these labs. You must be an advocate for yourself and request that your practitioner look deeper into your symptoms and, at the very least, rule out histamine intolerance. Not finding relief from your mysterious symptoms that can decrease your quality of life can be frustrating. The good news is that you can find relief with the targeted strategies listed in this book.

Western Treatments Don't Address the Root Cause of Histamine Intolerance

Even if histamine intolerance is diagnosed, no cure is available via Western medicine. Treatment involves dietary adjustments, antihistamines, H1-H4 receptor blockers (depending on symptoms), and mast cell stabilizing drugs. Keep in mind these all, with the exception of dietary modifications, address the symptoms only and don't get to the root of the condition. It is a pipe dream that these drugs will address the actual cause of your histamine intolerance since they are only masking symptoms.

The Risk of Antihistamines and H2 Antagonists

Once diagnosed, you may be tempted to reach for the easy solution in antihistamines (e.g., Zyrtec, Allegra, Benadryl) or H2 antagonist drugs (e.g., Zantac, Pepcid, Tagamet) to find relief, but in doing so, you may be making the problem worse by damaging your gut. Antihistamines and H2 antagonists block the production of stomach acid, which, over time, diminishes stomach acid and can lead to acid reflux. If you have been using these drugs regularly, you should consider restoring normal stomach acid production by taking betaine hydrochloride. Like most drugs, these options serve only as a bandage and do not address the root cause of your symptoms. In fact, suppressing the symptoms can make your body go to a deeper level to seek healing, which can make your symptoms worse, produce additional symptoms, and diminish your overall health and quality of life.

Stick to the Plan and Address the Root Cause

To address the source of histamine intolerance, you need to follow the plan outlined in this book, which includes minimizing dietary histamine, improving DAO activity, and reducing excess histamine production. Realistically, you need to get to the root cause of the histamine intolerance, which is frequently SIBO, mold, leaky gut, genetic mutations, mitochondrial dysfunction, some medications, or even gluten intolerance. The true cause of histamine intolerance almost always lies in the gut!

Take Control of Your Health and Beat Histamine Intolerance Naturally

The bottom line is that histamine intolerance is complex and tremendously complicated to diagnose. It is strongly recommended that you build a health-care team that includes a nutritionist experienced in food intolerance and the histamine contents of food and a histamine-intolerance-informed health-care practitioner. Lifestyle adjustments—managing stress, improving sleep, increasing physical activity, and reducing toxic load—are also critical. You are in control of your health and can make significant improvements in your symptoms based on your efforts. With time and a little guidance from informed health-care professionals, you can regain a high quality of life and say goodbye to the annoying symptoms of histamine intolerance.

REFERENCES

[1] Maintz L, Novak N. Histamine and histamine intolerance. *Am J Clin Nutr*. 2007 May;85(5):1185-96.

[2] De Zuani M, Del Secco C, Frossi B. Mast cells at the crossroads of microbiota and IBD. *Eur J Immunol*. 2018 Dec;48(12):1929-1937.

[3] Elieh Ali Komi D, Wöhrl S, Bielory L. Mast Cell Biology at Molecular Level: A Comprehensive Review. *Clin Rev Allergy Immunol*. 2020;58:342–365.

[4] Mukai K, Tsai M, Starkl P, et al. IgE and mast cells in host defense against parasites and venoms. *Semin Immunopathol*. 2016 Sep;38(5):581–603.

[5] Schwelberger HG. Histamine N-methyltransferase (HNMT) enzyme and gene. In: Falus A, editors. Histamine: biology and medical aspects. Budapest, Hungary: SpringMed Publishing, 2004: 53-9.

[6] Boudíková-Girard B, Scott MC, Weinshilboum R. Histamine N-methyltransferase: inhibition by monoamine oxidase inhibitors. *Agents Actions*. 1993 Sep;40(1-2):1-10.

[7] Schnedl WJ, Lackner S, Enko D, et al. Evaluation of symptoms and symptom combinations in histamine intolerance *Intest Res*. 2019;17:427–433.

[8] Maintz L, Bieber T, Novak N. Histamine intolerance in clinical practice. *Dtsch Ärztebl*. 2006;103:3477–3483.

[9] Wantke F, Proud D, Siekierski E, Kagey-Sobotka A. Daily variations of serum diamine oxidase and the influence of H1 and H2 blockers: A critical approach to routine diamine oxidase assessment. *Inflamm Res*. 1998;47:396–400.

[10] Schnedl W, Enko D. Histamine Intolerance Originates in the Gut. *Nutrients*. 2021 Apr; 13(4): 1262.

[11] Schnedl W, Enko D. Histamine Intolerance Originates in the Gut. *Nutrients*. 2021 Apr; 13(4): 1262.

[12] Comas-Baste OC, Sanchez-Perez S, Veciana-Nogues MT, et al. Histamine Intolerance: The Current State of the Art. *Biomolecules*. 2020 Aug; 10(8): 1181.

[13] Johnston CS. The antihistamine action of ascorbic acid. *Subcell Biochem*. 1996:25:189-213.

[14] Aguizdez JAG, Ayuso P, Cornejo-Carcia JA, et al. The Diamine Oxidase Gene Is Associated with Hypersensitivity Response to Non-Steroidal Anti-Inflammatory Drugs. *PLoS One*. 2012;7(11):e47571.

[15] Okutan G, Alcalde TP, Casares ER, et al. Cumulative effect of AOC1 gene variants on symptoms and pathological conditions in adult women with fibromyalgia: a pilot study. *Front Genet*. 2023 Jun 9:14:1180777.

[16] Arige V, Agarwal A, Khan AA, et al. Regulation of Monoamine Oxidase B Gene Expression: Key Roles for Transcription Factors Sp1, Egr1 and CREB, and microRNAs miR-300 and miR-1224. *J Mol Biol*. 2019;431(6):1127-47.

[17] Chen GL, Xu ZH, Wang W, et al. Analysis of the C314T and A595G mutations in histamine N-methyltransferase gene in a Chinese population. *Clin Chim Acta*. 2002 Dec;326(1-2):163-7.

[18] Turnbaugh PJ, Ley RE, Hamady M, et al. The human microbiome project. *Nature*. 2007 Oct 18;449(7164):804-10.

[19] De Palma G, Shimbori C, Reed DE, et al. Histamine production by the gut microbiota induces visceral hyperalgesia through histamine 4 receptor signaling in mice. *Sci Trans Med*. 2022 Jul;14(655):1895.

[20] Calam J, Bliss P, Murray S, et al. Histamine and Helicobacter pylori: are we closer to the answer? In: Hunt RH, Tytgat GNJ. (eds) *Helicobacter Pylori*. Springer, Dordrecht. 1998.

[21] Mou Z, Yang Y, Hall AB, et al. The taxonomic distribution of histamine-secreting bacteria in the human gut microbiome. *BMC Genomics*. 2021;22:695.

[22] Smolinska S, Winiarska E, Globinska A, et al. Histamine: A Mediator of Intestinal Disorders—A Review. *Metabolites*. 2022 Oct;12(10):895.

[23] Krell T, Gavira JA, Velando F, et al. Histamine: A Bacterial Signal Molecule. *Int J Mol Sci*. 2021 Jun;22(12):6312.

[24] Schink M, Konturek PC, Tietz E, et al. Microbial patterns in patients with histamine intolerance. *J Physiol Pharmacol*. 2018;69:579–593.

[25] Sanchez-Perez S, ComasBaste O, Duelo A, et al. Intestinal Dysbiosis in Patients with Histamine Intolerance. *Nutrients*. 2022;14(9):1774.

[26] Krell T, Gavira JA, Velando F, et al. Histamine: A Bacterial Signal Molecule. *Int J Mol Sci*. 2021 Jun;22(12):6312.

[27] Schnick M, Konturek, PC, Tietz E, et al. Microbial patterns in patients with histamine intolerance. *J Physiol Pharmacol*. 2018 Aug;69(4).

[28] Ogoburio I, Gonzales J, Shumway KR, et al. Physiology, Gastrointestinal. Available at: https://www.ncbi.nlm.nih.gov/books/NBK537103/. Accessed March 8, 2024.

[29] Guo FF, Yu TC, Hong J, et al. Emerging roles of hydrogen sulfide in inflammatory and neoplastic colonic diseases. *Front Physiol*. 2016;7:156.

[30] Dilek N, Papapetropoulus A, Toliver-Kinsky T, et al. Hydrogen sulfide: An endogenous regulator of the immune system. *Pharmacol Res*. 2020 Nov;161:105119.

[31] Lauritano EC, Gabrielli M, Scarpellini E, et al. Small intestinal bacterial overgrowth recurrence after antibiotic therapy. *Am J Gastroenterol*. 2008;103:2031–5.

[32] Kolkhir P, Balakirski G, Merk HF, et al. Chronic spontaneous urticaria and internal parasites--a systematic review. *Allergy*. 2016 Mar;71(3):308-22.

[33] Mukai K, Tsai M, Starkl P, et al. IgE and mast cells in host defense against parasites and venoms. *Semin Immunopathol*. 2016 Sep;38(5):581-603.

[34] Lu F, Huang S. The Roles of Mast Cells in Parasitic Protozoan Infections. *Front Immunol*. 2017; 8: 363.

[35] Ramsay DB, Stephen S, Borum M, et al. Mast Cells in Gastrointestinal Disease. *Gastroenterol Hepatol (N Y)*. 2010 Dec; 6(12): 772–777.

[36] Tanizaki Y, Komagoe H, Sudo M, et al. Candida-induced histamine release from basophils: relationship to house dust- and anti-IgE-induced secretion. *Acta Med Okayama*. 1985 Jun;39(3):191-7.

[37] Creasia DA, Thurman JD, Wannemacher RW Jr., et al. Acute inhalation toxicity of T-2 mycotoxin in the rat and guinea pig. *Fundam Appl Toxicol*. 1990;14:54–59.

[38] Capasso L, Longhin E, Caloni F, et al. Synergistic inflammatory effect of PM10 with mycotoxin deoxynivalenol on human lung epithelial cells. *Toxicon*. 2015;104:65–72.

[39] Amuzie CJ, Harkema JR, Pestka JJ. Tissue distribution and proinflammatory cytokine induction by the trichothecene deoxynivalenol in the mouse: Comparison of nasal vs. oral exposure. *Toxicology*. 2008;248:39–44.

[40] Liu C, Shen H, Yi L, et al. Oral administration of aflatoxin G1 induces chronic alveolar inflammation associated with lung tumorigenesis. *Toxicol Lett*. 2015;232:547–556.

[41] Kespohl S, Liebers V, Maryska S, et al. What should be tested in patients with suspected mold exposure? Usefulness of serological markers for the diagnosis. *Allergol Select*. 2022;6:118–132.

[42] Kritas SK, Gallenga CE, Ovidio CD, et al. Impact of mold on mast cell-cytokine immune response. *J Biol Regul Homeost Agents*. 2018 Jul-Aug;32(4):763-768.

[43] Kraft S, Buchenauer L, Polte T. Mold, Mycotoxins and a Dysregulated Immune System: A Combination of Concern? *Int J Mol Sci*. 2021 Nov; 22(22): 12269.

[44] Vyas S, Zaganjor E, Haigis MC. Mitochondria and cancer. Cell. 2016;166:555–566.

[45] Spinelli JB, Haigis MC. The multifaceted contributions of mitochondria to cellular metabolism. *Nature Cell Biol*. 2018 Jun 27;20:745-754.

[46] Picca A, Faitg J, Auwerx J, et al. Mitophagy in human health, ageing and disease. *Nature Metabolism*. 2023;5:2047-2061.

[47] Chelombitko MA, Chernyak BV, Fedorov AV, et al. The Role Played by Mitochondria in FcεRI-Dependent Mast Cell Activation. *Front Immunol*. 2020;11:584210.

[48] Zhang B, Alysandratos K-D, Angelidou A, et al. Human mast cell degranulation and preformed TNF secretion require mitochondrial translocation to exocytosis sites: relevance to atopic dermatitis. *J Allergy Clin Immunol*. 2011;127:1522–31.e8.

[49] Qian L, Nasab EM, Athari SM, et al. Mitochondria signaling pathways in allergic asthma. *J Investig Med*. 2022 Apr; 70(4): 863–882.

[50] Lieberman P. The basics of histamine biology. *Ann Allergy Asthma Immunol*. 2011 Feb;106(2 Suppl):S2-5.

[51] Zampeli E, Tiligada E. The role of histamine H4 receptor in immune and inflammatory disorders. *Br J Pharmacol*. 2009 May;157(1):24-33.

[52] Schnedl WJ, Lackner S, Enko D, et al. Evaluation of symptoms and symptom combinations in histamine intolerance. *Intest Res*. 2019;17:427–433.

[53] Diaz-Reixa JP, Rodriguez MA, Breijo SM, et al. Lower Urinary Tract Symptoms (LUTS) as a New Clinical Presentation of Histamine Intolerance: A Prevalence Study of Genetic Diamine Oxidase Deficiency. *J Clin Med*. 2023 Oct 31;12(21):6870.

[54] Schnedl W, Enko D. Histamine Intolerance Originates in the Gut. *Nutrients*. 2021 Apr; 13(4): 1262.

[55] Mušič E, Korošec P, Šilar M, et al. Serum diamine oxidase activity as a diagnostic test for histamine intolerance. *Wien Klin Wochenschr*. 2013;125:239–243.

[56] Manzotti G, Breda D, Di Gioacchino M, et al. Serum diamine oxidase activity in patients with histamine intolerance. Int. J. Immunopathol. Pharmacol. 2016;29:105–111. doi: 10.1177/0394632015617170.

[57] Steinbrecher I, Jarisch R. Histamin und kopfschmerz. *Allergologie*. 2005;28:85–91.

[58] Izquierdo-Casas J, Comas-Basté O, Latorre-Moratalla ML, et al. Low serum diamine oxidase (DAO) activity levels in patients with migraine. *J Physiol Biochem*. 2018;74:93–99.

[59] Rosell-Camps A, Zibetti S, Pérez-Esteban G, et al. Intolerancia a la histamina como causa de síntomas digestivos crónicos en pacientes pediátricos. *Rev Esp Enferm Dig*. 2013;105:201–207.

[60] Hrubisko M, Danis R, Huorka M, et al. Histamine Intolerance—The More We Know the Less We Know. A Review. *Nutrients*. 2021 Jul; 13(7): 2228.

[61] Komericki P, Klein G, Reider N, et al. Histamine intolerance: Lack of reproducibility of single symptoms by oral provocation with histamine: A randomised, double-blind, placebo-controlled cross-over study. *Wien Klin Wochenschr*. 2010;123:15–20.

[62] Kofler L, Ulmer H, Kofler H. Histamine 50-skin-prick test: a tool to diagnose histamine intolerance. *ISRN Allergy*. 2011 Feb 22:2011:353045.

[63] Wantke F, Gotz M, Jarisch R. Histamine-free diet: treatment of choice for histamine-induced food intolerance and supporting treatment for chronic headaches. *Clin Exp Allergy*. 1993 Dec;23(12):982-5.

[64] Music E, Silar M, Korosec P, et al. Serum diamine oxidase (DAO) activity as a diagnostic test for histamine intolerance. *Clin Transl Allergy*. 2011; 1(Suppl 1): P115.

[65] Raveendran VV, Tan X, Sweeney ME, et al. Lipopolysaccharide induces H1 receptor expression and enhances histamine responsiveness in human coronary artery endothelial cells. *Immunology*. 2011 Apr;132(4):578-588.

[66] Cimolai N. Comparing histamine intolerance and non-clonal mast cell activation syndrome. *Intest Res*. 2020 Jan;18(1):134–135.

[67] Kucher AN. Association of polymorphic variants of key histamine metabolism genes and histamine receptor genes with multifactorial diseases. *Russ J Genet*. 2019;55:794–814.

[68] Sanchez-Perez S, Celorio-Sarda R, Veciana-Nogues MT, et al. 1-methylhistamine as a potential biomarker of food histamine intolerance. A pilot study. *Front Nutr*. 2022 Oct 12:9:973682.

[69] Comas-Baste O, Latorre-Moratalla ML, Bernachhia R, et al. New approach for the diagnosis of histamine intolerance based on the determination of histamine and methylhistamine in urine. *J Pharm Biomed Anal*. 2017 Oct 25:145:379-385.

[70] D'Agostino L, Ciacci C, Daniele B, et al. Postheparin plasma diamine oxidase in subjects with small bowel mucosal atrophy. *Dig Dis Sci*. 1987 Mar;32(3):313-7.

[71] Maintz L, YU C-F, Rodriguez E, et al. Association of single nucleotide polymorphisms in the diamine oxidase gene with diamine oxidase serum activities. *Allergy*. 2011 Jul;66(7):893-902.

[72] Sanchez-Perez S, Comas-Baste O, Veciana-Noues MT, et al. Low-Histamine Diets: Is the Exclusion of Foods Justified by Their Histamine Content? Nutrients. 2021 May;13(5):1395.

[73] Sanchez-Perez S, Comas-Baste O, Costa-Catala J, et al. The Rate of Histamine Degradation by Diamine Oxidase Is Compromised by Other Biogenic Amines. *Front Nutr.* 2022 May 25:9:897028.

[74] Del Rio B, Redruello B, Linares DM, et al. The biogenic amines putrescine and cadaverine show in vitro cytotoxicity at concentrations that can be found in foods. *Sci Rep.* 2019 Jan 15;9(1):120.

[75] Parmentier R, Ohtsu H, Djebbara-Hannas Z, et al. Orexin/hypocretin and histamine: distinct roles in the control of wakefulness demonstrated using knock-out mouse models. *J Neurosci.* 2002;22:7695-711.

[76] Rehn D, Reimann HJ, von der Ohe M, et al. Biorhythmic changes of plasma histamine levels in healthy volunteers. *Agents Actions.* 1987 Oct;22(1-2):24-9.

[77] Swidsinski A, Dorffel Y, Loening-Baucke V, et al. Impact of humic acids on the colonic microbiome in healthy volunteers. *World J Gastroenterol.* 2017 Feb 7;23(5):885–890.

[78] Makrigianni EA, Papadaki ES, Chatzimitakos T, et al. Application of Humic and Fulvic Acids as an Alternative Method of Cleaning Water from Plant Protection Product Residues. *Separations.* 2022;9(10):313.

[79] National Health and Nutrition Examination Survey 2013-2014 Data Documentation, Codebook, and Frequencies Glyphosate (GLYP) - Urine (SSGLYP_H). Available at: https://wwwn.cdc.gov/Nchs/Nhanes/2013-2014/SSGLYP_H.htm.

[80] Samsel A, Seneff S. Glyphosate, pathways to modern diseases II: Celiac sprue and gluten intolerance. *Interdiscip Toxicol.* 2013 Dec;6(4):159–184.

[81] Theoharides TC, Tsolioni I, Ren H. Recent advances in our understanding of mast cell activation – or should it be mast cell mediator disorders? *Expert Rev Clin Immunol.* 2019 Jun;15(6):639–656.

[82] Samsel A, Seneff S. Glyphosate, pathways to modern diseases II: Celiac sprue and gluten intolerance. *Interdiscip Toxicol.* 2013 Dec;6(4):159–184.

[83] Hussain A, Saeed A. Hazardous or Advantageous: Uncovering the Roles of Heavy Metals and Humic Substances in Shilajit (Phyto-mineral) with Emphasis on Heavy Metals Toxicity and Their Detoxification Mechanisms. *Biol Trace Elem Res.* 2024 Feb 23. Online ahead of print.

[84] Stohs SJ. Safety and Efficacy of Shilajit (Mumie, Moomiyo). *Phytother Res.* 2014 Apr;28(4):475-9.

[85] K Jaiswal A, K Bhattacharya S. Effects of shilajit on memory, anxiety and brain monoamines in rats. *Indian J Pharmacol.* 1992;24:12–17.

[86] Carrasco-Gallardo C, Guzman L, Maccioni RB. Shilajit: A Natural Phytocomplex with Potential Procognitive Activity. *Int J Alzheimers Dis.* 2012;2012:674142.

[87] Keller JL, Housh TJ, Hill EC, et al. The effects of Shilajit supplementation on fatigue-induced decreases in muscular strength and serum hydroxyproline levels. *J Int Soc Sports Nutr.* 2019;16: 3.

[88] Pandit S, Biswas S, Jana BU, et al. Clinical evaluation of purified Shilajit on testosterone levels in healthy volunteers. *Andrologia.* 2016;48:570-75.

[89] Pingali U, Nutalapati C. Shilajit extract reduces oxidative stress, inflammation, and bone loss to dose-dependently preserve bone mineral density in postmenopausal women with osteopenia: A randomized, double-blind, placebo-controlled trial. *Phytomedicine*. 2022 Oct:105:154334.

[90] Cucca V, Ramirez GA, Pignatti P, et al. Basal Serum Diamine Oxidase Levels as a Biomarker of Histamine Intolerance: A Retrospective Cohort Study. *Nutrients*. 2022 Apr 5;14(7):1513.

[91] Neree AT, Pietrangeli P, Szabo PI, et al. Stability of Vegetal Diamine Oxidase in Simulated Intestinal Media: Protective Role of Cholic Acids. *J Agric Food Chem*. 2018;66(48):12657–12665.

[92] Neree AT, Soret R, Marcocci L, et al. Vegetal diamine oxidase alleviates histamine-induced contraction of colonic muscles. *Sci Rep*. 2020;10:21563.

[93] Comas-Baste I, Latorre-Moratalla ML, Sanchez-Perez S, et al. In vitro determination of diamine oxidase activity in food matrices by an enzymatic assay coupled to UHPLC-FL. *Anal Bioanal Chem*. 2019 Nov;411(28):7595-7602.

[94] Alemany-Fornes M, Boru J, Tintore M, et al. How reliable are DAO supplements? — A comparison of over-the-counter Diamine oxidase products. *BioRxiv*. 2023 Apr. Online ahead of print.

[95] Kettner L, Seitl I, Fischer L. Toward Oral Supplementation of Diamine Oxidase for the Treatment of Histamine Intolerance. *Nutrients*. 2022 Jun 24;14(13):2621.

[96] Kettner L, Seitl I, Fischer L. Evaluation of porcine diamine oxidase for the conversion of histamine in food-relevant amounts. *J Food Sci*. 2020 Mar;85(3):843-852.

[97] Manzotti G, Breda D, Di Gioachhino M, et al. Serum diamine oxidase activity in patients with histamine intolerance. *Int J Immunopathol Pharmacol*. 2016 Mar;29(1):105–111.

[98] Schnedl WJ, Schenk M, Lackner S, et al. Diamine oxidase supplementation improves symptoms in patients with histamine intolerance. *Food Sci Biotechnol*. 2019 Dec;28(6):1779–1784.

[99] Izquierdo-Casas J, Comas-Baste O, Latorre-Moratalla ML, et al. Diamine oxidase (DAO) supplement reduces headache in episodic migraine patients with DAO deficiency: A randomized double-blind trial. *Clin Nutr*. 2019 Feb;38(1):152-158.

[100] Yacoub MR, Ramirez GA, Berti A, et al. Diamine Oxidase Supplementation in Chronic Spontaneous Urticaria: A Randomized, Double-Blind Placebo-Controlled Study. *Int Arch Allergy Immunol*. 2018;176(3-4):268-271.

[101] Kovacova-Hanuskova E, Buday T, Gavliakova S, et al. Histamine, histamine intoxication and intolerance. *Allergol Immunopathol (Madr)*. 2015 Sep-Oct;43(5):498-506.

[102] Johnston CS. The antihistamine action of ascorbic acid. *Subcell Biochem*. 1996;25:189-213.

[103] Martner-Hewes PM, et al. Vitamin B-6 nutriture and plasma diamine oxidase activity in pregnant Hispanic teenagers. *Am J Clin Nutr*. 1986 Dec;44(6):907-13.

[104] Miyoshi M, Ueno M, Matsuo M, et al. Effect of dietary fatty acid and micronutrient intake/energy ratio on serum diamine oxidase activity in healthy women. *Nutrition*. 2017 Jul-Aug:39-40:67-70.

[105] Hamada Y, Shinohara Y, Yano M, et al. Effect of the menstrual cycle on serum diamine oxidase levels in healthy women. *Clin Biochem*. 2013 Jan;46(1-2):99-102.

[106] Martner-Hewes PM, Hunt IF, Murphy NJ, et al. Vitamin B-6 nutriture and plasma diamine oxidase activity in pregnant Hispanic teenagers. *Am J Clin Nutr*. 1986 Dec;44(6):907-13.

[107] Jarisch R, Wantke F. Wine and headache. *Int Arch Allergy Immunol*. 1996 May;110(1):7-12.

[108] Jarisch R, Weyer D, Ehlert E, et al. Impact of oral vitamin C on histamine levels and seasickness. *J Vestib Res*. 2014;24(4):281-8.

[109] Legleiter LR, Spears JW. Plasma diamine oxidase: a biomarker of copper deficiency in the bovine. *J Anim Sci*. 2007;85(9):2198-2204.

[110] Kehoe CA, Faughnan MS, Gilmore WS, et al. Plasma diamine oxidase activity is greater in copper-adequate than copper-marginal or copper-deficient rats. *J Nutr*. 2000;130(1):30-33.

[111] McGrath AP, Hilmer KM, Collyer CA, et al. The structure and inhibition of human diamine oxidase. *Biochem*. 2009;48:9810–9822.

[112] Nishida K, Uchida R. Role of Zinc Signaling in the Regulation of Mast Cell-, Basophil-, and T Cell-Mediated Allergic Responses. *J Immunol Res*. 2018 Nov 25:2018:5749120.

[113] Nishio A, Ishiguro S, Miyao N. Specific change of histamine metabolism in acute magnesium-deficient young rats. *Drug Nutr Interact*. 1987;5(2):89-96.

[114] Shalit M, Tedeschi A, Miadonna A, et al. Desferal (desferrioxamine)—a novel activator of connective tissue-type mast cells. *J Allergy Clin Immunol*. 1991;88:854–60.

[115] Roth-Walter F. Compensating functional iron deficiency in patients with allergies with targeted micronutrition. *Allergo J Int*. 2021 Apr;30:130-134.

[116] Pugin B, Barcik W, Westermann P, et al. A Wide Diversity of Bacteria from the Human Gut Produces and Degrades Biogenic Amines. *Microb Ecol Health Dis*. 2017;28:1353881.

[117] Schnedl WJ, Enko D. Histamine Intolerance Originates in the Gut. *Nutrients*. 2021;13:1262.

[118] Schink M, Konturek PC, Tietz E, et al. Microbial Patterns in Patients with Histamine Intolerance. *J Physiol Pharmacol*. 2018;69:579–593.

[119] Sanchexz-Perez S, Comas-Bste O, Duelo A, et al. Intestinal Dysbiosis in Patients with Histamine Intolerance. *Nutrients*. 2022 May;14(9):1774.

[120] Oksaharju A, Kankainen M, Kekkonen RA, et al. (2011) Probiotic Lactobacillus rhamnosus downregulates FCER1 and HRH4 expression in human mast cells. *World J Gastroenterol*. 2012;17(6):750-759.

[121] Kung HF, Lee YC, Huang YL, et al. Degradation of Histamine by Lactobacillus plantarum Isolated from Miso Products. *J Food Prot*. 2017 Oct;80(10):1682-1688.

[122] Dev S, Mizuguchi H, Das AK, et al. Suppression of Histamine Signaling by Probiotic Lac-B: a Possible Mechanism of Its Anti-allergic Effect. *J Pharmacol Sci.* 2008;107(2):159-166.

[123] Yu Z, Chen J, Liu Y, et al. The role of potential probiotic strains Lactobacillus reuteri in various intestinal diseases: New roles for an old player. *Front Microbiol.* 2023 Feb 1;14:2023.

[124] Liu Y, Alookaran J, Rhoads J. Probiotics in autoimmune and inflammatory disorders. *Nutrients.* 2018;10(10):1537.

[125] Koch RL, Pazdro R. Impact of Supplementary Amino Acids, Micronutrients, and Overall Diet on Glutathione Homeostasis. *Nutrients.* 2019 May;11(5):1056.

[126] Penissi AB, Rudolph MI, Piezzi RS. Role of mast cells in gastrointestinal mucosal defense. *Biocell.* 2003;27:163–172.

[127] Kempuraj D, Madhappan B, Christodoulou S, et al. Flavonols inhibit proinflammatory mediator release, intracellular calcium ion levels and protein kinase C theta phosphorylation in human mast cells. *Br J Pharmacol.* 2005;145:934–944.

[128] Li Y, Yao J, Han C, et al. Quercetin, Inflammation and Immunity. *Nutrients.* 2016 Mar; 8(3): 167.

[129] Uyanga VA, Amevor FK, Liu M, et al. Potential Implications of Citrulline and Quercetin on Gut Functioning of Monogastric Animals and Humans: A Comprehensive Review. *Nutrients.* 2021 Nov; 13(11): 3782.

[130] Llcek J, Jurikova T, Skrovankova S, et al. Quercetin and Its Anti-Allergic Immune Response. *Molecules.* 2016 May; 21(5): 623.

[131] Park HH, Lee S, Son HY, et al. Flavonoids inhibit histamine release and expression of proinflammatory cytokines in mast cells. *Drug Efficacy Safety.* 2008 Oct 29;31:1303-1311.

[132] Rakha A, Umar N, Rabail R, et al. Anti-inflammatory and anti-allergic potential of dietary flavonoids: A review. *Biomed Pharmacotherapy.* 2022 Dec;156:113945.

[133] Fu S, Ni S, Wang D, et al. Berberine suppresses mast cell-mediated allergic responses via regulating FcεRI-mediated and MAPK signaling. *Int Immunopharmacol.* 2019 Jun;71:1-6.

[134] Sun H, Wang H, Zhang A, et al. Berberine Ameliorates Nonbacterial Prostatitis via Multi-Target Metabolic Network Regulation. *OMICS.* 2015 Mar 1;19(3):186–195.

[135] Tian YJ, Li D, Ma Q, et al. Excess nicotinamide increases plasma serotonin and histamine levels. *Sheng Li Xue Bao.* 2013 Feb 25;65(1):33-8.

[136] Roschek Jr B, Fink RC, McMichael M, et al. Nettle extract (Urtica dioica) affects key receptors and enzymes associated with allergic rhinitis. *Phytother Res.* 2009 Jul;23(7):920-6.

[137] Roschek Jr B, Fink RC, McMichael M, et al. Nettle extract (Urtica dioica) affects key receptors and enzymes associated with allergic rhinitis. *Phytother Res.* 2009 Jul;23(7):920-6.

[138] Bakshaeee M, Pour AHM, Esmaeili M, et al. Efficacy of Supportive Therapy of Allergic Rhinitis by Stinging Nettle (Urtica dioica) root extract: a Randomized, Double-Blind, Placebo- Controlled, Clinical Trial. *Iran J Pharm Res*. 2017 Winter;16(Suppl):112-118.

[139] Din L, Lui F. Butterbur. Available at: https://www.ncbi.nlm.nih.gov/books/NBK537160/. Accessed March 7, 2024.

[140] Choi YW, Lee KP, Kim JM, et al. Petatewalide B, a novel compound from Petasites japonicus with anti-allergic activity. *J Ethnopharmacol*. 2016 Feb 03;178:17-24.

[141] Scheidegger C, Dahinden C, Wiesmann U. Effects of extracts and of individual components from Petasites on prostaglandin synthesis in cultured skin fibroblasts and on leukotriene synthesis in isolated human peripheral leucocytes. *Pharm Acta Helv*. 1998;72:376-378.

[142] Berger D, Burkard W, Schaffner W. Influence of Petasites hybridus on dopamine-D2 and histamine-H1 receptors *Pharm Acta Helv*. 1998;72:373-375.

[143] Thomet OAR, Schapowal A, Heinisch IVWM, et al. Anti-inflammatory activity of an extract of Petasites hybridus in allergic rhinitis. *Int Immunopharmacol*. 2002 Jun;2(7):997-1006.

[144] Lee DKC, Haggart K, Robb FM, et al. Butterbur, a herbal remedy, confers complementary anti-inflammatory activity in asthmatic patients receiving inhaled corticosteroids. *Clin Exp Allergy*. 2004 Jan;34(1):110-4.

[145] Mettler LG, Brecht K, Butterweck V, et al. Impact of the clinically approved Petasites hybridus extract Ze 339 on intestinal mechanisms involved in the handling of histamine. *Biomed Pharmacother*. 2022 Apr:148:112698.

[146] Zaghool SS, Shehata BA, Abo-Seif AA, et al. Protective effects of ginger and marshmallow extracts on indomethacin-induced peptic ulcer in rats. *J Nat Sci Biol Med*. 2015 Jul-Dec; 6(2): 421–428.

[147] Kawamoto Y, Ueno Y, Nakahashi E, et al. Prevention of allergic rhinitis by ginger and the molecular basis of immunosuppression by 6-gingerol through T cell inactivation. *J Nutr Biochem*. 2016 Jan:27:112-22.

[148] Hidalgo-Gutierrez A, Gonzalez-Garcia P, Diaz-Casado ME, et al. Metabolic Targets of Coenzyme Q10 in Mitochondria. *Antioxidants (Basel)*. 2021 Mar 26;10(4):520.

[149] Du Q, Meng W, Athari SS, et al. The effect of Co-Q10 on allergic rhinitis and allergic asthma. *Allergy Asthma Clin Immunol*. 2021 Mar 20;17(1):32.

[150] Deichmann R, Lavie C, Andrews S. Coenzyme Q10 and Statin-Induced Mitochondrial Dysfunction. *Ochsner J*. 2010 Spring;10(1):16–21.

[151] Singh A, D-Amico D, Andreux PA, et al. Direct supplementation with Urolithin A overcomes limitations of dietary exposure and gut microbiome variability in healthy adults to achieve consistent levels across the population. *Eur J Clin Nutr*. 202;76:297-308.

[152] D'Amico D, Andreux PA, Valdes P, et al. Impact of the Natural Compound Urolithin A on Health, Disease, and Aging. *Trends Mol Med*. 2021 Jul;27(7):687-699.

[153] Andreux PA, Blanco-Bose W, Ryu D, et al. The mitophagy activator urolithin A is safe and induces a molecular signature of improved mitochondrial and cellular health in humans. *Nature Metabolism*. 2019;1:595-603.

[154] Liu S, D'Amico D, Shankland E, et al. Effect of Urolithin A Supplementation on Muscle Endurance and Mitochondrial Health in Older Adults: A Randomized Clinical Trial. *JAMA Netw Open*. 2022;5(1):e2144279.

[155] Singh A, D-Amico D, Andreux PA, et al. Direct supplementation with Urolithin A overcomes limitations of dietary exposure and gut microbiome variability in healthy adults to achieve consistent levels across the population. *Eur J Clin Nutr*. 202;76:297-308.

[156] Uppada S, Zou D, Scott EM, et al. Paclitaxel and Urolithin A Prevent Histamine-Induced Neurovascular Breakdown Alike, in an Ex Vivo Rat Eye Model. *ACS Chem Neurosci*. 2022 Jul 20;13(14):2092-2098.

[157] Hu Y, Zhang L, Wei LF, et al. Liposomes encapsulation by pH driven improves the stability, bioaccessibility and bioavailability of urolithin A: A comparative study. *Int J Biol Macromol*. 2023 Dec 31;253(Pt 7):127554.

[158] Kim HM, Cho Sh. Lavender oil inhibits immediate-type allergic reaction in mice and rats. *J Pharm Pharmacol*. 1999 Feb;51(2):221-26.

[159] Seo YM, Jeong SH. [Effects of Blending Oil of Lavender and Thyme on Oxidative Stress, Immunity, and Skin Condition in Atopic Dermatitis Induced Mice]. *J Korean Acad Nurs*. 2015 Jun;45(3):367-77.

[160] Mitoshi M, Kuryama I, Nakayama H, et al. Effects of essential oils from herbal plants and citrus fruits on DNA polymerase, cancer cell growth inhibitory, anti-allergenic, and antioxidant activities. *J Agric Food Chem*. 2012 nov;60(145):11343-50.

[161] Shinde UA, Kulkarni KR, Phadke AS, et al. Mast cell stabilizing and lipoxygenase inhibitory activity of Cedrus deodara (Roxb.) Loud. Wood oil. *Indian J Exp Biol*. 1999 Mar;37(30:258-61.

[162] Pathak MP, PAtowary P, Das A, et al. Beta caryophyllene exerts its anti-allergic potency by inhibiting histamine release and pro-inflammatory markers in mast cells. *Proc Annual Meeting Japanese Pharmacol Soc*. 2018 Jan.

INDEX

heparin, 8, 10
histamine decarboxylase (HDC) gene, 33
histamine liberators, 35-36
histamine N-methyltransferase (HNMT), 11, 13, 14, 33, 67
histamine receptor H1 (HRH1) gene, 33
homocysteine, 13, 51, 59
humic acid, 38-40
hydrogen-dominant SIBO, 16-17
Hydrogen sulfide-dominant SIBO, 17

I

immunoglobulin E (IgE), 11, 19, 21, 30, 32, 39, 56, 63, 65, 68, 69
interleukins, 32, 39
iron, 47, 48, 50, 52, 53, 54

K

kaempferol, 64
Klebsiella pneumoniae, 55

L

Lactobacillus bulgaricus, 57
Lactobacillus casei, 57
Lactobacillus plantarum, 56
Lactobacillus reuteri, 56
Lactobacillus rhamnosus, 14, 56
Lactobacillus saerimneri, 57
lavender, 38, 71, 72
leaky gut, 15, 20, 74
lemon, 71, 72
leukotrienes, 10, 67, 71
lipopolysaccharide, 32
luteolin, 64

M

magnesium, 39, 47, 49, 50, 53, 54, 59
mast cell activation syndrome, 19, 32-33

mast cells, 8-10, 11, 19, 21, 23, 26, 29, 32, 35, 39, 46, 50, 56, 63-72, 73
methane-dominant SIBO, 16-17
1-methylhistamine, 34
methylation, 11, 13, 51, 57-61, 65
microflora, 39, 55
migraine, 7, 13, 20, 27, 45-46, 67
mitochondria, 14, 17, 21-23, 41, 69, 70, 74
mitophagy, 23, 70
mold, 19-21, 74
mold allergies, 20
mold mix 1, 21
mold toxicity, 20, 21
monoamine oxidase B (MAO-B), 11
monoamine oxidase (MAO) gene, 13, 33
methylenetetrahydrofolate reductase (MTHFR), 13, 33, 51, 57-61
Mycoplasma pulmonis, 30
mycotoxins, 20-21, 41
myricetin, 64

N

neuromodulators, 9
neurotransmitters, 7, 9, 13, 14, 26, 48, 58, 65
NSAIDs, 12, 13

O

organic cation transporter 3 (OCT3), 67
overmethylation, 57, 58, 59, 60, 61

P

parasites, 15, 18-19
peppermint, 18, 71, 72
phosphorus, 47, 49, 53
PrimaVie, 40, 41
prostaglandins, 10, 21, 32, 66

protozoans, 18
Pseudomonas aeruginosa, 14, 30
putrescine, 13, 36

Q
quercetin, 44, 63-64, 66

R
respiratory, 9, 20, 21, 27
rutin, 64

S
S-adenosyl-L-methionine (SAMe), 11, 13, 51, 58, 59
sauerkraut, 7
seasonal allergies, 7, 58, 59, 67, 73
serine, 60-61
serotonin, 8, 9, 16, 26, 58, 59, 65
shilajit, 40-42
single nucleotide polymorphisms (SNPs), 12, 28, 33
skin-prick test, 29-30
sleep, 13-26, 36-38, 42, 58, 74
small intestinal bacterial overgrowth (SIBO), 15-18, 19, 22, 74
small intestinal fungal overgrowth (SIFO), 19
spermidine, 36

spermine, 36
SSRI antidepressants, 58, 59
stem cells, 26
stinging nettle, 66
systemic mastocytosis, 29

T
T cells, 7, 8, 26
tart cherry extract, 37-38
tele-methylhistamine (t-MH), 11
Th1/Th2 balance, 63
toxins, 13, 19, 20, 21, 38, 39, 41
tyramine, 36

U
undermethylation, 57-60
urolithin A, 70-71, 72

V
vagus nerve, 9
vitamin B6, 47-48, 52, 60
vitamin B12, 47, 51, 55
vitamin C, 12, 44, 47, 48, 52, 54, 55, 60

Z
zinc, 39, 47, 49, 50, 52, 53-54, 59
zonulin, 15

www.ingramcontent.com/pod-product-compliance
Lightning Source LLC
Chambersburg PA
CBHW070813280326
41934CB00012B/3175